THE SILVER CLOUD DIET

Sustainable Eating for the 21st Century

Whole and Unprocessed Foods

For Health, Weight Control, and Long Life

2nd edition, new information, more recipes

By

Dr. John Salerno, Board Certified Family Practice

Complementary Medicine

And

Linda West Eckhardt

James Beard Award winning cookbook author

I would like to thank the many people in my life who have been so important to me in creating this book.

First, my wife Helene and my seven year old son, John, and 3 year old daughter, Sophia, have always been there for me and have lent their unconditional support and love. Helene is a dedicated wife, mother, and chef who continues to always inspire and encourage my work.

My children now remind me what is bad for me to eat. John is an avid cyclist who rides with me every morning rain or shine. It is on these special rides where I have received perhaps the best insight for my book from a child's perspective.

Sophia, the aspiring 3 year old artist and dancer has given me ideas for the importance of developing healthy tastebuds at an early age and is also quick to remind me to give her daily vitamins.

I would like to thank my brother Louis for his always brilliant advice and caring. He has given me the inspiration and shown me the work ethic I needed to be successful.

I would also like to thank my wonderful parents John and Louise who have always nurtured me with love and support beyond words. Aunt Josie was my inspiration to take vitamins at a early age and is always there for me.

Lastly, my best friend and cousin Vinny whose friendship and support from childhood has and will always be valuable.

Dr. John Salerno

The Silver Cloud Diet by Dr. John P. Salerno and Linda West Eckhardt

Photography by Gwendolen F. Cates

Published by Madison Lexington Books, New York, New York
http://www.thesilverclouddiet.com

ISBN: 978-0-615-41549-9

Printed in the United States of America

Books are available in quantity discount for colleges, churches, organizations or other groups in conjunction with services, keynotes, or products offered or alone. For more information please email sales@thesilverclouddiet.com.

The Salerno Center
161 Madison Av. #7SW
New York, NYC, NY 10017
Ph: (212) 582-1700

This book is intended solely for informational and educational purposes and not as personal medical advice. Please consult your doctor if you have any questions about your health.

Table of Contents 4

Now You Can Finally Do it

Preface by Dr. John P. Salerno

What Makes The Silver Cloud Diet Sustainable?

And how is it different from other low carb diets? Isn't it just Atkins all over again?

These questions come to my office often. Some people like the idea that it's Atkins, others not so much. So what is the deal, anyway?

I owe an enormous debt of gratitude to the late, great Dr. Robert Atkins who was my boss, my mentor and my friend. I worked in his office as a young doc and saw with my own eyes the value of the protocols he developed – first to help people with heart disease, then, almost as if by accident, it turned out that these protocols helped people lose weight.

What did Atkins really say? He believed that a low carb diet could help treat heart disease, and help people lose weight. He was right.

But things have changed since I started out in his office. I'm talking about the food supply.

In the last twenty years, the food supply in the United State has degraded. And as the food supply has gotten worse, the obesity and other lifestyle ailments, including diabetes, heart disease, cancer, and Alzheimer's have gotten much, much worse.

It's as if our very environment has become poisoned. The food, the water, the air.

In order to save our own lives and the planet, we must adopt sustainable practices at the table. This means understanding that our health depends on sustainable agriculture products and practices, and public policy that supports health.

Last summer, we went to D.C. to testify before the U.S.D.A. about the upcoming Food Pyramid. We said there what we believe, that industry has corrupted the process and made recommendations to Americans that do not support health.

Now, we are encouraged to note that a significant body of scientists have signed on to form a committee agreeing with our position, that Americans must be provided with a safer, more nourishing food supply. Our very lives depend on it. There are so many issues that can interfere with our health and well being.

This fact was brought home to me, up close and personal, when I volunteered at ground zero after 9-11. I began treating people who had volunteered to help in the dreadful task of picking through the rubble, hunting for survivors after the attack on The World Trade Center.

Some of those hapless souls have become my patients, and I have cared for them ever since.

So what can the ordinary person do to protect himself? Eat organic produce. Choose wild caught fish, and grass fed beef. Drink filtered water (and not from a plastic bottle). Purify the air in your home if you live in a polluted area.

These precautions will help to normalize your weight, improve your health, and make for a long and glorious middle age. If Dr. Atkins were alive today, he would know, even more, the huge task we have ahead of us, to improve the health of Americans.

We must exercise our true power in the market place. Reject GMO foods, industrial farming, and confined animal feeding operations. We will get what we demand in the market and we can provide a healthier dinner table for ourselves and our children just by being aware of what we put into our mouths.

Yours in good health,

Dr. John Salerno

THE TOP TEN QUESTIONS ABOUT THE SILVER CLOUD DIET

1. How is this diet different from Atkins?
2. What can I eat in a restaurant?
3. Road food, office food, eating on the run?
4. I'm worried about not eating vegetables in the detox phase.
5. Where can I find appropriate food?
6. Will I ever be able to eat a piece of cake?
7. I don't want to prepare a separate meal for myself. What about my partner? My children?
8. How much weight can I expect to lose?
9. When do I go off the diet?
10. Tell me one more time. Why should I eat fat?

When Dr. Atkins developed his protocols some 30 years ago, the food supply was less degraded than it is now. Unfortunately, due to the increase in processed foods, junk foods, and our degraded farm land, the Atkins protocols just won't work any more.

You have to take a more proactive stand to preserve your health and weight. I find with my patients, that their body needs a period of rest from the assaults of the Western Diet and so a short period, say 2 weeks, of complete relief from carbohydrates of all types will make it possible to change your life, reset your body clock, and put you on the road to health and long life.

This is the good news. Even in the Detox phase of the diet, you can eat out. Take the burger out of the bread, skip the French fries and enjoy it. Eat grilled fish, roast chicken, pot roast, tenderloin of pork, shrimp, scallops, pates. Any of these work fine in a restaurant at any phase of the diet.

Plan ahead. Boil eggs and keep them on hand for car trips, office snacks, lunches on the run. Lay in a supply of jerky, salmon, nuts of any kind, string cheese. Any of these nutrient dense foods will keep you satisfied and on track.

The notion that we have to eat vegetables every day is new. Even as recently as a hundred years ago, mankind only had vegetables during the growing season. To go for a short period with no vegetables is natural and healthy and actually rests your body.

Man has been on this earth for thousands of years. We've only eaten the same foods 12 months a year for about 100. Don't worry. Give your body a rest. The Detox will take 5 to 15 pounds off, reduce your waist size, and more importantly rest your overstressed liver and pancreas.

We recommend buying food as "close to the ground" as possible. In the grocery store, choose organic produce, eggs, and dairy. At the farmer's market, ask the vendors how they grow their crops. Find a local provider for meats and fish if possible.

As your health becomes more vigorous, and you lose weight, and increase your activities, beginning with a walking regimen of 10,000 steps a day, yes, you will be able to eat more carbohydrates, even the occasional piece of cake.

Please don't prepare a special meal for yourself. Everyone in the family should be eating a broad and varied diet of unprocessed foods. Your partner and children may kick about it, but if you retain a positive attitude, they will come on board and every one of you will be healthier.

I have patients who are thrilled to lose 20 pounds. I have patients who have lost upwards of 200 pounds with no pills and no pain, just learning to love a broad and varied diet of unprocessed foods.

You are not going "off" the diet ever. You are making decisions to take care of your body by eating great food for the rest of your life. And if you ever feel your weight creeping back up, give yourself a week of Dr. Salerno's Detox and you'll reset your clock and be back on target in no time.

And remember that natural fat is the most nutrient dense food there is. It is the lubricant of your joints, and the element that makes your brain work best. It keeps your hair shiny and your skin unwrinkled.

Once you remove the unhealthy processed carbohydrates from your diet, you don't need to worry about natural fat. And perhaps the best part of eating plenty of natural fat is that it is nature's appetite suppressant. Pay attention to your body and your body will take care of you.

A word from Linda Eckhardt

When I met John Salerno, I had fallen into a pit that I ascribed to the fact that I write about food, test recipes day in and day out, am constantly thinking about food, and quite simply, love my work. The net result was that I was about 30 pounds overweight, OK, truth time – 40 pounds, beginning to have trouble with my knees, and not as energetic as I had been in the past.

At first, I believed John's ideas were pretty radical. I knew he had been a protégé of Dr. Atkins and had a number of patients who had regained their health while losing the weight following his recommendations, but to tell you the truth, I didn't think I could do it.

I couldn't quite imagine a diet that started off with nothing but high natural animal fat, meat, fish and eggs and little else – what John calls the Full Fat Fast. It sounded absurd to me.

Who would do such a thing? But I consented to have my blood drawn and tested and the results were alarming. I had elevated blood sugars and insulin resistance, high cholesterol, high blood pressure, and a stunning shortage of vitamin D. How would eating nothing but meat and eggs do anything but make that worse?

But I have a friend, Angela Phelan, also a food professional, and about my age, who recommended Dr. S. to me. About 10 years ago, she had a heart attack and surgery to put in stents. Taking all the medicines recommended by her cardiologist, she quickly developed diabetes type II and was told she'd spend the rest of her life pricking her finger.

But she's a sensible Italian girl with a long history of eating what could be described as the Mediterranean diet and she knew what the diabetes docs were telling her sounded like nonsense.

Dr. Atkins was still alive then, and she went to see him. At that time, Dr. Salerno was his junior doc in the office, and between them, they put her on a course of only real food, traditionally prepared, not unlike what she and Dr. Salerno had both experienced in their Italian American childhoods.

Angela, with Robert Atkins and John Salerno's help became one of the early standard bearers in the movement sometimes known as "Slow Food", or the "Green Movement", or "Sustainable Cuisine."

My friend got well. She lost 40 pounds. She hasn't pricked her finger in more than nine years. The type 2 Diabetes vanished. And now, at the tender age of 72, she remains a highly capable and fully employed food professional who flies all over the country overhauling commercial kitchens and menus for clients as diverse as some of America's top universities and private schools, to business and government dining rooms.

May I tell you she is converting the institutions of America to her new **Fresh and Natural Café** concept and is having enormous success getting people back into school and office dining rooms again. She gets hired to consult in these big kitchens because management often finds that they suffer low usage by workers and students. Sometimes, as few as 15% of them will eat in the facility's dining room.

They call on Angela to help them improve their bottom line, get the workers and students back at the table. After inspecting these facilities, here's what she recently reported to the execcutives for one corporation

"The reason no one will eat here is because you are serving them shit." This is the blunt truth she tells these execs on the first meeting after observing dining rooms with steam tables and deep fryers and workers who do nothing but microwave and heat processed foods. "You want people to eat in your dining room, you gotta give 'em real food."

Angela is, of course, building on the good work of Alice Waters who is revolutionizing school lunch room programs based on the same principles.

People in this country are beginning again to demand real food. No matter where they are eating. Corporate America is beginning to get the picture. Public schools are getting the picture And not a minute too soon.

We all have the power to change the food that's offered to us. Demand organic produce and your grocer will provide it. Call for grass fed meats. Even the big box sores and clubs are beginning to carry it. Anybody checked a Walmart superstore lately? You'll be pleasantly surprised. You get what you demand and the prices will come down.

Back to my initial experience with Dr. Salerno. He explained to me that we needed to shock my system by removing all carbohydrates from my diet. I freely confess to a love for all things sweet and sugary.

In my past life, if I could combine fat, sugar, and flour – in any of a million iterations – I was happy. In fact, it is fair to say that I was addicted to these combinations. Some of my most successful books are based on these combinations: two bread books, a dessert book, and a cake book. I told myself that bread was the staff of life and how could that be bad?

The way my knees were beginning to feel, bread was not only a staff but perhaps I might also need a crutch. People in the food business do a lot of standing in one place, tense, hunched over hot stoves and chopping blocks. If you're pouring a lot of overly processed carbs down your gullet because they taste good and give you a quick rush, then you're on your way to perdition as surely as the cocaine addict in the corner office.

I decided to give Dr. Salerno's plan a try. For two weeks, I did as I was told. I aimed for 1000 calories a day. I ate an omelet every morning – and boy did I get creative with the combinations. I started off buying a new All-Clad 8-inch pan, and a scale to weigh the food.

Sometimes I ate bacon or sausage too. He told me that following breakfast, I should eat four additional meals of 2 ounces of natural fat and protein spaced out over the day. So about three hours after the omelet, I'd have a snack, then later I'd eat a 2 ounce hamburger, or a piece of steak, or a pork chop, or a can of sardines, or salmon. For snacks, I might eat some full fat cheese, or nuts, or foie gras, or pate, or pork skins.

You get the idea. If it was protein and it was full of natural animal fat, I could eat it.

About the third day I began to notice a change. I had a rush of energy. I was no longer tired all the time. I was never hungry and desperate to wolf down a bunch of cookies or a plate of pasta.

After two weeks, the change was noticeable. I had lost 12 pounds. My waist had gone down 2 inches. My hair was shiny. My eyes were bright . Even my skin seemed to be more supple. And, best of all, I could once again work the way I did 15 years ago.

My only complaint was constipation, and my cookbook writing partner, Diana Butts, provided an easy solution to that. Eat 2-3 tablespoons of shirataki noodles daily (sold often as Miracle Noodles) which are pure indigestible fiber and your troubles are over.

So when I went back for a check up, we drew blood again, checked my blood pressure, and began the next phase.

Now here is where Dr. Salerno began to talk in terms I really understood. He knows the typical American diet is unhealthy. He told me that if he could snag 100 people walking the streets of New York City, he was sure at least 80 of them would have elevated blood sugars and insulin resistance.

Eating empty calories, overly processed foods, and junk food have predictable results: overweight, a steady march towards diabetes, heart disease, stroke, cancer, and Alzheimer's.

I told him I was worried because high blood pressure runs in my family, and my mother died of a stroke. Not something I ever want to happen to me.

And there were even more concerns that I had. When I mentioned cholesterol, he went on, "Cholesterol levels are only a minor player if at all in the risk for heart disease or stroke! Some studies have deduced that elevated cholesterol is a result of a heart attack, in other words, it's the body's response to the insult. Not a cause, but a result."

But what can we do? I asked. Do what our grandmothers did, he answered, eat real food. And that's when I knew he was singing my song. I've been writing for twenty five years that there's more about nutrition that we don't know than we do, and your best shot to a long and healthy life is a diet made up of a broad and varied selection of whole, unprocessed foods, free from chemical or hormone interference. I just conveniently forgot that flour and sugar where part of that processed food equation.

Now, in our world today real, unprocessed foods have been hard to come by with our reliance on industrial food production, factory farmed meats and fish, genetically modified seed, chemically altered food products, and overly processed faux-foods made to taste like something by ingenious tricks devised in some so-called Dr. Frankenstein food lab.

But, as John Salerno and I both know. The tide is turning. A movement has begun. Farmer's Markets are springing up all over the country. The locavore movement is taking hold. Slow Food Nation is gaining converts by the day.

People are beginning to rebel against cruel, inhumane treatment of farm animals. Victory gardens are popping up in people's yards. Artisan farms are springing up growing everything from tomatoes to geese to sheep and hogs and cows. They're making artisan cheeses and sausages and all manner of products the old fashioned way with no chemicals or preservatives. I even took all the grass up and turned my entire backyard into a vegetable garden.

If you read Gary Taubes <u>Good Calories, Bad Calories,</u> and Michael Pollan's <u>In Defense of Food</u>, you will see that rational thought has moved the goal posts and we may even be playing a different game. We're all on the same page. Eat real food. Avoid the fake and the faux foods and your health will improve.

John Salerno and I are building on the good work of Taubes and Pollan who have presented sound scientific treatises on the state of the Western Diet today. Our concept is that we will offer a work of applied science, a clinical treatise that will show people how to put the information to use in their everyday lives.

We decided we would write this book together that would help people to normalize their weight and live a long and vigorous life. Together, we present the fruits of our labors, two years and many long discussions with and tests by us and John's patients. We wish you health. We wish you a long and vigorous life.

Take the first step and you'll be on your way.
And by the way, the third round of blood and lab work I had showed some estimable improvements. Blood sugars in the normal range. No more need for all those blood pressure pills I've been swallowing for fifteen years. No more vitamin deficiencies.

Most surprising to me was the change in my eyes. I knew I couldn't see well in my eyeglasses but I had no way of knowing, until my ophthalmologist told me that the normalizing of my blood sugars had substantially improved my eyesight. Who knew?

This way of life is going to work for me as well as it did for my grandmother who lived on the ranch, ate beef steak every day of her life and worked in her garden well into her eighties. As John Salerno told me on that day, "you've added 20 years to your lifespan by making these simple changes."

It wasn't hard. I promise. You can do it too. Stay with us and we'll lead the way.

Why You Need to Read This Book

The United States is on the verge of a health crisis of monumental proportions. We may have virtually eradicated polio, measles and other devastating diseases, made childbirth significantly safer for both mothers and infants and saved countless lives with antibiotics.

Likewise, dramatically lower rates of infectious diseases including tuberculosis, rheumatic fever, influenza and periodontal disease mean that today's children, unlike their peers 70 years ago, can expect to survive beyond than their first few years.

However, these and other impressive medical victories are now being undermined by a bevy of other health problems, many of our own making. For the first time, children born today are likely to have a shorter lifespan than their parents, thanks to damage that will be wrought by the terrible trio of obesity, diabetes and Alzheimer's.

Our genes undeniably play a role in our health and longevity; nonetheless, up to 80 percent of disease is the result of environmental forces.

I use the term "environmental" in the broadest sense to include lifestyle choices we can control, such as what we eat, whether we consume alcohol or smoke, how physically active we are, even the household products we use, as well as those largely beyond our control—including but not limited to industrial toxins in the air and water and pesticides that contaminate and weaken the soil.

We are beginning to pay the price for our disregard for the environment, not just in terms of global warming—devastating as that is—but also in our own health and that of our children.

The facts are:

- The actual life span of Americans who survive infancy has not changed in more than 60 years. Sixty-five percent of American adults are overweight or obese.
- Diabetes has become epidemic in the United States and is on the rise throughout the world.

Even as our bodies are burdened with an increasingly greater toxic burden, we are less able to defend ourselves against assault, weakened as we are by the standard American diet. And now we are exporting this unhealthful way of eating to the rest of the world.

The multiple reasons for the decline in our overall health, as reflected by these facts:

- There are more than 100,000 chemicals in regular use in the United States, with an additional seven new ones approved every day.
- Infants are born with almost 300 chemicals in their blood.
- Our bodies contain hundreds of toxins, including some—such as DDT—that were banned 30 years ago.
- Common pesticides and other chemicals that mimic hormones are implicated in the sharp rise of genital abnormalities in infants and low sperm counts in men.
- According to the U.S. Geological Survey, in a 2002 study of stream water samples, 69 percent contained detergents and 66 percent contained disinfectants. The oceans—and their fish—are contaminated with heavy metals and other toxins.
- Our factory farm raised meat and dairy products are laced with growth hormones and antibiotics. Much of the soil in which crops are grown is depleted of vital nutrients such as calcium, phosphorus, iron, selenium, chromium, and riboflavin.

Therein lies a double whammy: Not only is our air, water, and soil—increasingly toxic, but our food supply, which would normally protect our bodies from toxins, lacks the nutrients to do the job. To compound the problem, our diet is increasingly dominated by foods without much nutritive value—other than calories—fast foods, especially foods full of white flour, sugar, and other refined carbohydrates, as well as trans fats which may actually do more harm than good as a diet staple.

Most industrialized countries have eliminated hunger as a public health problem, only to have it replaced with another dangerous condition: obesity.

And ironically, people who subsist on doughnuts, bagels, cheeseburgers, potato chips, pizza, soft drinks and other junk food may be undernourished even though they are well upholstered.

The truth is that obesity and starvation are two sides of the same coin.

According to one Harvard study, the average American eats only 3 servings of vegetables and fruit a day, a mere 1-1/2 cups, while 9 servings or 4-1/2 cups are optimal. Shortchanging the diet in such a serious way means missing out on the natural sources for many vitamins and minerals.

Ironically, most of the diseases that plague us in the 21st century are associated with excess consumption—specifically heart disease, diabetes, obesity, many forms of cancer and even Alzheimer's. Excess intake of white flour, sugar, other refined carbohydrates, and trans-fats are the culprits that rob us of our health, stamina, and life span.

Nutrition continues to be the stepchild of the medical establishment, which focuses instead on treating illness after the fact, usually with expensive drugs—each with its long list of side effects—rather than prevention.

This, despite the fact that statistics published by the American Medical Association show that 73 percent of all diseases are directly related to nutrition.

Meanwhile, the drug industry is in peak health, stimulated by "expanding markets" for new "products." Government agencies and health organizations like the American Cancer Society routinely state that the causes for most of the disease they represent are "unknown."

And so the elephant in the living room continues to go unmentioned. This conscious blindness of the role of the diet and the environment is akin to a refusal to acknowledge the reality of global warming.

The evidence cannot be ignored. Men's average sperm count has declined by about one-third over the last 30 years. A male resident of the United States is eight times more likely to die of prostate cancer than a man in Japan.

We have treated our planet like a garbage dump and now the toxins are coming home to roost—in our bodies and the bodies of our unborn children. It turns out that when a person experiences genetic damage as a result of a toxin, the defective gene can be passed on to our children and grandchildren.

The prognosis may sound grim, but I firmly believe there is a solution, and a relatively simple one at that. The very technology that has polluted our planet can also provide us with the know-how to undo past mistakes and avoid similar ones in the future.

There is a tremendous body of research on the processes and chemicals that weaken the body and allow disease to take hold, as well as the role that nutrients play in fortifying the body against disease or even turning back the process of disease. We can harness that knowledge to counter both environmental assaults and genetic weaknesses.

Because I have satellite practices in Japan and Brazil in addition to The Salerno Center in New York, I have the opportunity to compare a culture that has been industrialized for three quarters of a century with ones that until recently were primarily rural. All too many of my foreign patients now suffer from the same diseases that have plagued Americans for decades, strongly suggesting environmental influences.

My understanding of the healing power of nutritious food and the health risks inherent in refined and processed foods was honed working side by side with the late, great Dr. Robert C. Atkins.

Many of his long-term patients are now my patients and I can see the impact that his dietary approach has had on their health. Many are getting on in years but are still remarkably vigorous and free of disease, due, no doubt to decades of following his low-carb, high-nutrient protocol, all clinically validated in their medical records.

Drawing upon my own clinical experiences in nearly 20 years in family practice and those of other complementary physicians, as well as a vast body of medical research, I have developed a strategy to dramatically regulate your weight, decrease your chances of developing cancer, heart disease, diabetes or other devastating diseases.

By putting only good food and water into your body and regularly removing toxins, you can, to a large extent, take charge of your health and live a long, vital and vigorous life.

We call it **The Silver Cloud Diet**.

My goal in this book is to show you how making some simple but profound changes in your daily life can dramatically boost your chances for remaining—or becoming—healthy, despite the toxic soup in which we stew. Against such a challenge, three squares and a daily multivitamin won't give you the defensive edge you need.

The Silver Cloud Diet is a proactive approach to nutrition based on a high protein, high natural fat, low-carbohydrate, low-glycemic diet, fortified with nutritional supplements targeted to strengthen your immune system, reduce inflammation, and destroy free radicals that cause dangerous oxidization.

I also advocate regular detoxification to cleanse your body of accumulated poisons in your liver and kidneys.

Of course, to ensure good health and longevity, keep your weight under control, drink plenty of pure water, engage in regular physical activity and find ways to deal with stress.

That's not to say that fate can't play its cruel tricks. Just as a careful and conscientious driver can still be injured in a traffic accident through no fault of his own, you can take good care of yourself and still have the misfortune to develop a serious illness.

What I am saying is this: If you take good care of yourself—and I will tell you how to do so—you can vastly improve your odds of living a long healthy life. I can't promise that you will live to be 85, 90, or even 100, be immune to all disease and remain active and alert until you die peacefully in your sleep of old age.

However, I can give you the tools to dramatically decrease your *risk* of dying from cancer, heart disease or stroke or spending your last decades as a victim of diabetes, Alzheimer's, respiratory failure or another chronic disease—and increase your chances of aging gracefully, sound in body and mind.

So, yes, if you take responsibility to use the tools I will give you, you can profoundly impact your destiny.

Now you can finally do it.

Yours in good health,

Dr. John P. Salerno

Introduction

Dr. John Salerno and Linda West Eckhardt's **The Silver Cloud Diet** is a scientifically proven program that helps people lose weight safely and fast. It challenges conventional wisdom on diet, weight control and disease. And the diet, a lifestyle plan, offers added benefits: immediate results and radically changed blood chemistry. Adult-onset (Type II) diabetes can be stopped in its tracks, which in turn reduces the risk of a heart attack, stroke, Alzheimer's and Parkinson's diseases.

The diet is based on eating real unprocessed foods with plenty of fat and protein to regulate bodily functions, control hunger, and prevent cravings.

The diet controls insulin levels so the body can properly burn sugars, rather than store them as fat, particularly in the midsection, the so-called belly fat.

And best of all, there is no need for calorie counting. Once the reader begins to understand portions, they get to choose from a healthy assortment of meat, fish, eggs, full fat cheeses, oils, nuts.

The body will begin to regulate itself normally and they can begin to enjoy most vegetables, fruits, and even small amounts of complex carbohydrates, like whole grains and certain sweets.

This is not as radical as it may first appear. Traditional cultures worldwide and over time have practiced what we're teaching now. Whole, unprocessed foods, grown close to home, cooked in simple ways, produce meals that taste good and nourish the body and the soul.

A healthy ration of natural animal fats, including generous portions of saturated fats, have been proven in numerous studies since the 1920's to have salutary effects on everything from brain function to cancer.

So what happened? Over the past thirty years Americans have been bombarded by an industrial food industry that threw out these common sense notions and turned the family farm into a feedlot.

This in turn led to a depletion in the quality of animal meat as well as the soil itself. Then the pharmaceutical industry stepped in, offering up an ever more complicated array of "solutions" to all the ills that followed, including the introduction of food-like substances in ever growing portions that neither nourish nor satisfy.

Together these industries have been telling Americans that low fat diets were best for their health. That is, quite simply, a lie.

You can see the result on any street in America today. We are the fattest of the Western countries, and, for the first time in history, have a generation of people who may not live as long or as healthily as their grandparents.

The Silver Cloud Diet protocol addresses these issues. Weight can be normalized. Diners can enjoy food as it was meant to be enjoyed, in the company of friends and family.

People who accept the tenets of this revolutionary plan will no longer look at food as medicine, or something to be endured. They will relish their meals, because they'll be eating real food, well prepared, and served with joy.

Children's lives can be saved by making a conscious choice right now to stop buying junk food, eating in fast food restaurants, and stuffing their innocent mouths with fake food that can doom them to lives with diabetes, high blood pressure, and, perhaps cancer and heart disease.

Dr. Salerno's patients, some of whom began with Dr. Robert Atkins, are living proof that one can eat plenty of natural fats, protein, wholesome vegetables, fruits, nuts and grains prepared in time-honored methods ad live long and vigorous lives. And the bottom line is it is an easy protocol to follow - there is no pain or punishment involved.

The Silver Cloud Diet can save lives and change the way America eats, one person at a time.

How the Diet Works

It's a fair guess that if you've been eating the normal American diet two things have happened: your weight has crept up and your energy has gone down.

Dr. Salerno and Linda West Eckhardt want to make one thing clear. It's not your fault you're fat. To have lived in this country for the past thirty years was to be pelted with more fake facts, fake foods, and fake science than any time in the history of mankind. But readers can turn that around, starting with this book.

If you walked into a doctor's office now complaining that you're overweight, a good doctor would test your blood to see if you had elevated blood sugar, also known as blood glucose.

Your blood glucose level in considered normal if it's below 100, but if your numbers were between 100 and 125, it's fair to describe your condition as prediabetic, and over 125 can be considered diabetes.

If you are at least fifteen pounds overweight, it's a good guess that your blood glucose levels are over the normal reading.

If your blood glucose levels are over 100, your body has made a serious maladaption to a diet with too many processed carbohydrates and sugars. Your cells, which rely on the energy released by the glucose that is made from the normal digestion process, may not be able to process that glucose because you have become insulin resistant.

Insulin is a hormone produced by the pancreas that unlocks the glucose for use by the cells in your body. All energy, whether for movement, thinking, or building your body, depends on a balance between the glucose produced by your digestion and the insulin released by your body.

But things get out of whack when you take in too many over-processed carbs. Glucose goes up and down wildly throughout the day. Eat cold cereal or a bagel for breakfast, and you may find yourself famished an hour or so after you ate.

Some people with severe insulin resistance will get clammy and sweaty. Their heart may pound. All these are symptoms of blood glucose levels that have become unstable, (hypoglycemia).

We gain weight because insulin becomes elevated from a diet loaded with high carbs: high fructose corn syrup, white flour, sugars, soda pop, all the places where these diet busters are hidden in the prepared foods we buy. All of these enemies tell the body to store fat.

To regain control of your bodily functions, you need to shock your system by removing all carbohydrates for a short period – about two weeks. We call this the *Full Fat Fast*. This isn't as hard as it sounds, and the results will astound.

By following this simple plan, Dr. Salerno has seen patients lose anywhere from 5 to 15 pounds. They will discover, on about day three, that their energy level suddenly zooms up.

Within two weeks, their skin will begin to glow, their hair will begin to shine, and even their nails will grow faster.

They won't suffer that mid-afternoon slump when all you want is a nap. Their clothes may feel suddenly loose, and if the reader measures their waist, they'll see it's gone down a couple inches.

If people give the Dr. Salerno's Detox: *Full Fat Fast* a chance they will have begun the road to excellent health and optimum weight. In this phase, we subscribe five small meals each day, with full fats.

The dieter is going to eat nothing but real food, preferably organic meats, fish, poultry, sausages, full fat cheeses, and eggs. People may have to change the way they shop and start visiting their local farmer's markets and whole food stores because the days of eating chemically laden, hormone-laced fake foods are over.

Bouts of constipation can be stopped by eating fiber rich Miracle Noodle (shirataki), about 3 tablespoons with meals or as a snack with a carb free salad dressing, just drops really.

Once people move to the next phase – what we call *The Marathon*, they'll be eating a broad and varied array of organic and whole meats, fish, poultry, eggs, vegetables, fruits, and grains. This is a traditional diet, not unlike one that was practiced in countries around the world before the advent of industrial farming.

What people won't be eating are so-called "health" or diet foods, and certainly no overly processed foods. You will be eating real food, and your body will be grateful. At this point making a conscious effort to up your fat intake will yield remarkable results. Your weight will go down, your blood chemistry will improve, and your waist size will shrink.

But fat will make me fat, won't it?

No, it won't. The reason your weight is elevated is that your body has converted glucose in your body to stored fat because it's been confused by the normal American diet which is loaded with sugars, processed carbohydrates, and in many cases, junk food.

On the other hand, Dr. Salerno has treated people who believed they were doing the healthiest thing possible by becoming vegetarians or vegans, and yet their bodies didn't lie. Some were overweight. Their blood glucose was elevated. Some had full blown diabetes type 2, when all they had done was eat vegetables and fruits, and some even stuck to all organic produce. How could this have happened?

Some vegetables and many fruits are nature's sugars. While fruits and vegetables have high nutrient values, they will overwhelm our already stressed systems and produce insulin resistance, particularly the wrong kinds, like corn and peas, carrots, pineapples, grapes and watermelon.

It's easy to understand this when you consider that any seed in nature must, by design, be packed with sugars so that the seed can develop. But these need to be avoided at least at first for people who wish to change their life and improve their health.

When readers begin *The Marathon*, at first they'll be restricted to green, leafy vegetables and the cruciferous vegetables (for example, arugula, bok choy, broccoli, Brussels sprouts, cabbage, cauliflower, collard greens, mustard greens, radishes, and watercress).

Vegetables that grow underground should be avoided at first: onions, parsnips, carrots, potatoes: all the root vegetables which are, by their very nature, high sugar.

If there's one thing we know, the human body is amazingly resilient, and if you just give it half a chance, it can and will recover. Dr. Salerno has seen it in his office for more than 20 years of medical practice, dealing with patients whose weight was completely out of control.

He has treated patients successfully who had failed on many other diets: low fat, a range of gimmicky one-ingredient diets (grapefruit, avocado, cabbage et al), Weight Watchers, Jenny Craig. Most of these low fat diets are doomed to fail, whereas this plan puts these patients on the right track for a new way of life.

People can change. And the secret they'll quickly discover is this: you will never be hungry on this diet. You will never feel that faint, clammy, desperate feeling that signals hypoglycemia again because your body will have plenty of energy at the ready stored from a steady supply of fat in the diet to get you through the day. You'll be eating real food.

The Atkins Connection

Thirty years ago Dr. Robert Atkins, Dr. Salerno's mentor and friend before his death, introduced to the world the concept of low carbs and its positive effect on weight loss. His diet worked for millions of people who lost weight and gained energy.

However, after inheriting the Atkins Center patients and continuing Dr. Atkins' work, Dr. Salerno is seeing many patients today have difficulty losing with Atkins induction. approach. Why is this?

The food supply in America has changed for the worse since Robert Atkins did his ground breaking work thirty years ago. There are more empty foods, more junk foods, more fast foods, and more fake foods than Robert Atkins ever could have imagined. It's as if we had forgotten what real food looks like or tastes like.

All of Dr. Salerno's patients are required to do a glucose tolerance test with insulin, and he notes recently a very striking and consistent phenomenon.

Many more patients have exceedingly high insulin levels which remain stuck. It's a direct result of today's society eating too many sugars and refined carbohydrates, including many hidden sugars in processed foods (such as high fructose corn syrup, which appears in almost every prepared food in the marketplace today). It is truly insidious and dangerous.

And if that weren't enough, the modern eater must read labels zealously. Dr. Salerno recently picked up a bottle of cranberry juice cocktail which proudly trumpeted that it contained no high fructose corn syrup.

But the fine print revealed that after water, cane sugar was the next ingredient. This sort of three card monte in the food business tends to confuse Dr. Salerno's patients and the world.

Today, as a result of the difference in foods offered in the market place, patients can't lose weight on Atkins Induction like they did thirty years ago.

During this same period, people have stopped cooking from scratch, have begun eating out more often – some statistics say that people eat out more than 50% of the time, and when they buy foods in the market place, they tend to be the so-called "value added" prepared food products.

This means there are so many hidden sugars, carbohydrates, and chemicals in the diets of most Americans that they don't even know what they're putting into their mouths much of the time.

It is only when Dr. Salerno places them on a regimen of high fat and no carbs that we can see a decrease in insulin with the resulting weight loss. As mentioned before, we call this the *Full Fat Fast* phase of the diet. It prepares patients for the long range change in their eating habits we call *The Marathon*.

Sometimes his patients are afraid of this phase of the plan, thinking that it's unhealthy not to eat vegetables. Dr. Salerno reminds them that mankind has only had vegetables year round for a limited time in the scheme of history, and that ancient man routinely went through the winter with no vegetables or fruits at all.

> *Our bodies have a deep and ancient understanding of a fat fast – it's how mankind was able to survive. Trust your body. It often knows better than you do what you need.*

Complex carbohydrates are then reintroduced slowly, beginning with leafy vegetables, and later, berries, beans and seeds, and finally whole grains. This isn't hard and represents a giant leap backwards to the wisdom of our forebears who ate almost no processed foods and were lean and healthy for most of their lives.

The modern Western diet that has dominated our choices in the market has created poor eating habits in the population and a rise in health problems. We know from experience that The Silver Cloud Diet will interrupt this cycle and change lives.

Slow Food Nation

The tide is turning. A movement has begun. Farmer's Markets are springing up all over the country. The locavore movement is taking hold. Slow Food Nation is gaining converts by the day. People are beginning to rebel against cruel, inhumane treatment of farm animals. Victory gardens are popping up in people's yards. Artisan farms are springing up growing everything from tomatoes to geese to sheep and hogs and cows. They're making artisan cheeses and sausages and all manner of products the old fashioned way with no chemicals or preservatives.

Why I recommend Organic Foods To My Weight Loss Patients

Because I want my patients to eat nutrient dense foods, you have to begin with the dirt. The overuse of pesticides, herbicides, and other chemical additives for the growth of monoculture genetically modified crops, including corn, soy, sugar beets, rice, canola, and others have wreaked havoc with the soil.

These grain and bean crops grown in this sterile soil are used not only to create overly processed foods, but are the basis for animal feed that is fed to factory farmed meats and farm raised fish. The results are food products with empty calories, unknown long term health effects, and almost certain capacity for making people fat.

Why is this? The ancient wisdom of mankind says you should eat until you are satisfied, and these foods simply don't satisfy us. Add to that the chemicals added to the so-called value-added foods which are put there to replace the natural goodness that has been lost and you have a real problem.

These food additives, with unpronounceable names and unknown derivatives are known categorically as excitotoxins. Did you ever wonder why Dad could sit down in front of the television to watch the ball game and eat an entire package of corn chips?

It's the Dr. Strangelove additions designed in the lab to make that food so tasty, Dad's natural satiety switch is turned off. In the food labs, these additives are known as *excitotoxins.*

Those added chemicals, which by the way, even s. on fresh produce that isn't organic by way of sprays and dip. chemical baths, can derail any weight loss program.

Chemicals can increase food cravings, cause water retention, and can actually cause weight gain. These same additives are often allergenic, and can cause insulin to spike, playing havoc with those people who are pre-diabetic, or diabetic.

When I go back to Italy, where my family is from, I am amazed at how much better the food tastes. Europe does not permit genetically modified crops, or, as a rule, does not support factory farming. Therefore, you can see with your own eyes and taste for yourself the fact that fewer people are overweight, and the food just plain tastes better.

But I am encouraged because a food revolution has begun in this country and people are demanding a more humane treatment of animals, are rejecting high fructose corn syrup, soy products made from genetically modified seed, and are calling for locally grown food products, the so-called locavore movement.

In an article I contributed to in January 2010, Men's Health magazine, I have discussed the cholesterol problem and shown how saturated fat and carb avoidance increase LDL particle size and decrease risk for heart disease and stroke.

Some of my patients have asked why I don't support a vegetarian diet, given the risks of eating factory farmed meat. The answer to that can be seen in the test tube. I've had numerous vegetarian and vegan patients who had elevated blood sugars, type 2 diabetes, and other health problems.

The answer which I propose is to eat a nutrient rich diet made up of plenty of saturated fat, protein, and fruits and vegetables which are organic, grass fed, and wild caught. (see www.thesilverclouddiet.com)

I get a lot of surprised looks from my patients when I tell them to eat more saturated fats to lose weight. They will start in telling me they've been eating a low fat diet for years. But they don't make the connection between this diet and their health problems, including overweight, type 2 diabetes, memory problems, and arthritis.

I explain to them that the body must have saturated fats for proper brain function, cell development, and satiety. Plus it just makes people look better. Fat carries flavor and makes people feel full and satisfied quicker.

I can spot the low fat high carb dieter in a moment. Dry skin, wrinkles, and broken fingernails. Those are the telltale signs that show. Lab work reveals many more.

So I propose that people eat adequate natural saturated fat, protein, and organically grown fruits and vegetables for optimum health and weight maintenance. It works for my patients.

Health Issues: The Silver Cloud Lifestyle Plan addresses the concerns of the overweight and the obese.

Obesity and The Metabolic Syndrome

The metabolic syndrome is comprised of five risk factors that dramatically increase the likelihood of developing diabetes, as well as coronary artery disease, stroke, hypertension and Alzheimer's. Each condition is in itself a risk for diabetes and cardiovascular disease, but en masse, they vastly compound the likelihood of serious disease. You need have only three of these five conditions to be diagnosed with the metabolic syndrome:

- Truncal obesity. In men, this means a waist of 40 inches or more; in women, 35 inches or more.
- Hypertension, meaning blood pressure of 135/85 mmHg or higher.
- High triglycerides, meaning 150 mg/dL or more.
- Low HDL ("good") cholesterol, meaning less than 40 mg/dL for men and less than 50 mg/dL for women.
- High fasting blood sugar, meaning 110 mg/dL or higher.

About 44 percent of Americans over the age of 50 has the metabolic syndrome, also known as prediabetes.

Metabolic Syndrome Leads to Dementia and Alzheimer's

According to the latest studies, there is no end in sight for the increasing rise in metabolic syndrome among Americans. As more and more people become overweight and obese, the hard numbers for metabolic syndrome rise at an alarming rate.

And perhaps the worst part of the news is that even children are demonstrating this condition, due to poor diet and inactivity.

Metabolic syndrome is actually a collection of risk factors for type 2 diabetes and heart disease that includes abdominal obesity (belly fat) high blood pressure, elevated blood sugar, low HDL (good) cholesterol, and high triglycerides.

Researchers believe more that while 50 million Americans had metabolic syndrome in 1990, and that number has skyrocketed to 64 million today and is beginning a geometric progression that will result in a huge number of Americans with heart disease and cognitive disorders in their old age.

The largest numbers of subjects sowing metabolic syndrome are young women. Actually younger and younger.

But we see this as an opportunity to help people understand why low carb diets, taken on at an early age can prevent the deadly slide from metabolic syndrome to diabetes type 2, heart disease, Alzheimer's and dementia.

This worldwide problem is being studied in laboratories from Australia, to England, to the United States with many other countries including Japan in between.

Prospectively, it is a problem than an individual can handle quite easily. Choose a healthy low carb diet, like the Silver Cloud, get exercise and your chances for suffering this long slide into senility is greatly reduced.

For prevention and treatment of Alzheimer's and dementia, we teach people to eat a diet high in saturated fats and proteins from grass fed meats and wild caught fish. We show them why they must avoid sugars, and processed carbs of all kinds. We have a long list of patients on our roster who are doing much better on this regimen.

One of the interesting counter-intuitive things we have shown is that you are not what you eat, but rather what your body does with what you eat. Eating saturated fat does not make you fat and lead to the dreaded metabolic syndrome. Eating processed carbohydrates does.

Laboratory studies of blood samples shows that subjects who eat a low fat diet which is always high carb, actually have worse fats in their bloodstream, than those who eat a low carb, high dietary fat diet.

We know from experience that not only do people lose weight, but their overall health improves on our low carb regimen. Keeping blood glucose and insulin under control bodes well for a long and healthy life.

PREVENTING AND TREATING TYPE 2 DIABETES

Mrs. T came to my center suffering from moderate obesity and type 2 diabetes. She was taking nearly 100 units of insulin and was on Glucophage, a drug used to lower glucose levels. She was having difficulty losing weight, her blood sugars still averaged around 170, she was tired all the time and depressed. She was only 48 years old.

When she first came to the Salerno Center extensive blood tests were taken as well as a fasting and 2 hours after eating a high carb meal, insulin and glucose were taken. Mrs. T's insulin levels were through the roof as were her glucose levels. Her thyroid gland was underactive, she had a huge amount of candida in her blood and her triglycerides were extremely elevated, so typical for diabetics. Her blood pressure was also high. This poor women was a stroke or heart attack waiting to happen.

I placed Mrs. T immediately on a low carb, yeast free diet where most cheeses, vinegar & mushrooms were eliminated. She was placed on Salerno Glucose Factor and Salerno Multi vitamin; Anti Aging Factor as well as probiotic for yeast and Salerno Blood Pressure Factor to lower her elevated blood pressure. She was also given a good amount of fish oils to lower her triglyceride level. Triglyceride elevation is much more problematic for stroke and heart disease especially in woman than cholesterol levels. The fish oils were also given to decrease her blood thickness which was also found to be elevated.

She was also placed on a thyroid medication. Her insulin injections were reduced to accommodate her new diet and vitamins. After one week Mrs. T lost 4 pounds, her insulin requirement decreased another 15%. Mrs. T was feeling more energetic and less depressed. She lost another 4 pounds the following week and continued to reduce her insulin to nearly ¼ of what she begun with. By week 16 Mrs. T was completely off her insulin and had lost 36 pounds. She hadn't felt this great in years and was now beginning a running program. Mrs. T's tryglycerides had normalized, her blood pressure was perfect and by week 48 was even off her glucophage medication.

Cases like these number in the hundreds at the Salerno Center. A modified version of the diet and supplementation program could cut the risk of Type 2 diabetes by over 95% in the general population.

Diabetes Mellitus, both types 1 and 2, are diseases that prevent your body from properly using the energy from the food you eat. Diabetes Type 1 occurs when the pancreas (an organ behind your stomach) produces little insulin or no insulin at all.

Type 2 can be thought of as a lifestyle disease which occurs because an improper diet and lack of exercise creates a situation wherein the pancreas makes insulin, but the insulin does not work as it should. This condition is called insulin resistance.

Often, I find my patients confuse type 1 and type 2 diabetes. Type 1 diabetes, also known as juvenile diabetes can develop at any age, but it most commonly appears in children, adolescents and young adults and is a result of a malfunctioning pancreas. Type 2 results from a pancreas that has been exhausted by a bad diet and lack of exercise.

One of the most alarming epidemics in our country is Type 2 diabetes, which even now, reaches into the childhood population to inflict its deadly consequences. This is one malady which can be linked inextricably to our Western diet and life of inactivity. On the flip side, it is one ailment that is almost completely preventable, provided you take a proactive stance against it.

PROTECT AND PREVENT

The following strategies will help reduce your risks for Type 2 diabetes:

- Know whether you have a family history of the disease.
- Lose weight if you are overweight (a BMI of more than 24.9).
- Exercise for a minimum of half an hour most days of the week.
- Don't drink alcohol in excess or at all if you have problems with unbalanced blood sugar.
- Obtain most of your carbohydrates from fresh, organic vegetables and some fruit and whole grains.
- Supplement your diet with recommended nutrients.
- After age 45, have your blood sugar levels checked at least every three years.

Ballooning rates of Type 2 diabetes have become an indictment of our lives of inactivity, over-consumption as well as a reliance on sweets and other junk foods full of empty carbohydrates. The US is ranked third in the number of cases of diabetes in the world—although it is the top ranked western/industrialized nation. Here are some facts from the International Diabetes Federation:

- Type 2 Diabetes affects more than 230 million people worldwide and is expected to affect 350 million by 2025.
- In 2003, the five countries with the largest numbers of people with diabetes were India (35.5 million), China (23.8 million), the United States (16 million), Russia (9.7 million) and Japan (6.7 million).
- By 2025, the number of people with diabetes is expected to more than double in Africa, the Eastern Mediterranean and Middle East, and South-East Asia, and rise by 20% in Europe, 50% in North America, 85% in South and Central America and 75% in the Western Pacific.
- Each year a further 7 million people develop diabetes.
- Each year over 3 million deaths are tied directly to diabetes. Every 10 seconds a person dies from diabetes-related causes.
- Diabetes is the fourth leading cause of death by disease globally.
- At least 50% of all people with diabetes are unaware of their condition. In some countries this figure may reach 80%.

People with diabetes are two to four times more likely to develop cardiovascular disease (CVD) than people without diabetes. Cardiovascular disease is the number one cause of death in industrialized countries. It is also set to overtake infectious diseases as the most common cause of death in many parts of the developing world. For each risk factor present, the risk of cardiovascular death is about three times greater in people with diabetes as compared to people without the condition.

One-third of American children born in the year 2000 are predicted to develop Type 2 diabetes. Even developing countries are seeing the incidence of diabetes skyrocket. China and India are now vying for the dubious distinction of having the largest number of diabetics in the world, as economic growth and newfound prosperity has lead to the adoption of Western eating habits and reduction in physical labor.

In both societies, where malnutrition was long rampant, being plump and idle were traditionally seen as status symbols; today, in both countries obesity is fast becoming a public health issue among segments of the population.

The association of diabetes with affluence in such countries is in stark contrast with the United States, where diabetes is more common among the poor.

Defining Diabetes

At its most simple, diabetes is a disorder of the glucose metabolism. In plain English, this means that you have diabetes when your body is unable to quickly and efficiently deal with blood sugar (glucose) produced from the breakdown of carbohydrates and other foods.

Consider the classic American dinner of macaroni and cheese casserole with a side salad. The noodles, cheese, milk-based sauce and breadcrumbs are full of carbohydrates along with fat and protein. The salad vegetables contain more carbohydrates, as does the salad dressing—along with fat.

The starchy carbohydrates in the noodles and bread crumbs begin to break down into glucose almost the minute you put them in your mouth—the salad vegetables take longer to turn to glucose—and the process is completed in your digestive system. (Protein and fat break down more slowly).

Your body functions within a fairly narrow blood sugar level range, so as highly processed carbohydrate foods begin to convert to glucose and your blood sugar level rises, your pancreas releases the hormone insulin.

The job of insulin is to ferry blood sugar from your blood stream to your cells, where it can be converted to energy. Any extra blood sugar is converted to glycogen and stored in the liver and muscle cells for use at a later date.

When the glycogen storage areas are full, the remaining glucose is stored as body fat. With fuel for immediate energy needs, plus two auxiliary storage areas—glycogen for the short term and body fat for the long term—this backup system allowed early man to survive for reasonably long periods when food was in short supply.

Feast or Famine

Obviously, things have changed over the millennia. For most of us, the closest we ever get to a period of famine is the 12 or so hours between dinner and breakfast.

Nor do we expend vast amounts of energy traveling everywhere by foot tracking game and trying to keep warm without central heat. . Too many carbs will tax your pancreas. And that can lead to diabetes II.

Let's look at the sequence of events that lead to diabetes.

Step 1: Insulin Resistance

The typical diet in the United States and increasingly in other industrialized countries consists of an excessive number of calories, often in the form of processed food—meaning primarily refined carbohydrates, which quickly convert to glucose.

As long as you continue eat this way, your body never needs to burn its fat for energy. The first sign that diabetes may be in your future is with your expanding waistline. Most people see extra pounds as a cosmetic issue, but they can also gradually make you insulin resistant.

That means that your cells are less responsive to the effects of insulin. It is important to state that not everyone with insulin resistance is overweight; nor is everyone who is overweight becoming insulin resistant, but the two are often associated. Why insulin resistance happens is not completely understood but inflammation appears to play a role.

Step 2: Insulin Resistance with Hyperinsulinism

Because insulin is less effective in making the cells take up the glucose and thereby normalize the blood sugar level, the pancreas releases more of it, resulting in elevated levels of insulin in the bloodstream.

Instead of the normal rise and fall of both blood sugar and blood insulin levels that occur after a meal, the balance has been disturbed. An individual now has both insulin resistance and hyperinsulinism, meaning that after each high-carbohydrate meal, glucose levels rise, prompting a large spike in insulin.

Step 3: Insulin Resistance, Hyperinsulinism and Low Blood Sugar

As time passes, the mechanism linking insulin and blood sugar becomes increasingly inefficient. It takes longer for the pancreas to produce insulin after a meal and then it overproduces, causing the blood sugar level to drop precipitously when a heavy dose of insulin finally kicks in.

The result, called reactive hypoglycemia, or low blood sugar, can kick off a number of symptoms such as peaks and valleys in energy, jitters, irritability and even brain fog. Cravings for sweets and other carbohydrate foods are also common as the body tries to elevate its blood sugar.

Step 4: Prediabetes

Step 3 can go on for years, but eventually the delay in insulin response, causes blood sugar levels to begin to peak above the normal range. The rollercoaster ride now becomes even wilder.

Two hours or so after a high carbohydrate meal, the blood sugar level is higher than it should be, often provoking sleepiness.

Then the insulin level spikes, resulting in the symptoms of low blood sugar described above. This trio of conditions—insulin resistance, hyperinsulinism and impaired glucose tolerance—is considered prediabetes.

Step 5: Type 2 Diabetes with Insulin Resistance and High Insulin Production

Eventually, although the pancreas continues to overproduce insulin, it no longer works in a timely fashion, resulting in dangerously high postprandial (after a meal) blood sugar levels.

Step 6: Type 2 Diabetes with Little or No Insulin Production

Eventually, unless intervention occurs, the beta cells of the pancreas become dysfunctional and can no longer churn out insulin or produce inadequate amounts. In addition to elevated postprandial blood sugar levels, fasting blood sugar levels (at least eight hours after a meal) are also in the danger zone.

According to the American Diabetes Association, a diagnosis of diabetes includes a fasting blood sugar of 126 mg/dL or higher on two readings and a postprandial reading of 200 mg/dL or higher after a high carbohydrate meal on two occasions.

It is not until this point that many people find out that they have diabetes, often as a result of a host of symptoms that can include increased thirst, hunger and the need to urinate. Weight gain and blurred vision are other symptoms.

A Worldwide Epidemic

The process that leads to Type 2 diabetes can take years, but it does not necessarily proceed slowly. When you consider how most people eat and the fact that two-thirds of American adults are overweight or obese, it could seem that most of the population is likely to develop diabetes.

Although the situation is dire, it is not quite that bad. Some people have a built-in propensity to blood sugar and insulin imbalances and others do not. If you have such a propensity but never trigger it with overeating and eating the wrong kind of food, you may never know you have such an inclination.

That said, there is no question that diabetes has reached epidemic proportions. Just how bad is it? In the United States, almost 21 million people, including children, or 7 percent of the population has diabetes, although almost one-third of them are unaware that they have the disease.

Another 41 million have pre-diabetes. Most children have Type 1 diabetes, which is the result of a lack of insulin caused by the destruction of beta cells in the pancreas, but increasingly more children have Type 2, or diabetes mellitus, which used to be called adult-onset diabetes.

This chapter focuses on Type 2 diabetes, which is preventable and to a certain extent reversible with lifestyle changes.

The United States is hardly alone in its diabetes epidemic. In Europe, 7.8% of the adult population, over 48 million adults, were estimated to have diabetes in 2003.

Type 2 diabetes is on the increase, not just in the United States, Europe, China and India, but also in many other countries where social and economic changes are occurring, such as the Republic of Korea, where by 1990 7.9 percent of the population had been diagnosed with diabetes, up from just 1.5 percent in 1971.

About 7.5 percent of New Zealanders have diabetes, as do as many as 10 percent of Maoris. Residents of Hong Kong, Japan and Singapore also have especially high rates.

Diabetes is a devastating disease all by itself, accounting for roughly 224,000 deaths in the United States alone each year and an estimated 3 million worldwide.

Terrible as these statistics are, diabetes is also intimately linked to a number of other serious or life-threatened conditions, including heart disease, stroke, high blood pressure, kidney disease, blindness, amputations of digits or limbs, diseases of the nervous system, gum disease, sexual dysfunction and complications of pregnancy, and ultimately Alzheimer's.

ASSESSING YOUR RISKS

A family history of diabetes is a clear message that you face an increased risk for the disease, along with several other matters beyond your control, but many critical factors are in your hands.

Age, Gender, and Race

Although Type 2 diabetes increasingly strikes children and young adults, it is far more common in older people, particularly after age 45. Almost 21 percent of Americans aged 60 and older have diabetes.

Men are slightly more likely than women to get the disease, although African-American, Hispanic, Native American, Asian American and Pacific Islander women are at least two to four times more likely than non-Hispanic white women to develop it.

Black Americans who do not have a Hispanic background are 1.8 times more likely to have diabetes than non-Hispanic whites. The same figure applies to residents of Puerto Rico.

Mexican Americans are not far behind, being 1.7 times more at risk than non-Hispanic whites. Native Americans fare even worse—2.2 times more likely than non-Hispanic whites.

Adult Hawaiians, whether natives or of Asian or Pacific islands descent, are more than twice as likely to have diabetes than whites. Asian Americans living in California are at slightly less risk: 1.5 times that of non-Hispanic whites.

Surplus Pounds

I know I sound like a broken record, but as with numerous other diseases, being overweight increases the odds of developing diabetes. Being overweight—meaning a BMI above 24.9—is the biggest risk factor for Type 2.

The younger a woman is when she puts on extra pounds, the more likely it is that she will wind up as a diabetic. On the flip side, when women lose weight and keep it off, they can reduce their risk.

When overweight gives way to obesity—meaning a BMI of 30 or more—the risk rises exponentially.

As with cardiovascular disease, where a person carries weight is significant. Apple-shaped men and women, who have thick waists—what doctors call truncal obesity—are more prone to diabetes than pear-shaped folks, who are heavy in the hips and buttocks.

For Women Only

Two conditions associated with the female reproductive system are also linked to the development of diabetes. If a woman has had what is called gestational diabetes during pregnancy (it goes away after she gives birth) or has given birth to an infant who weighed more than nine pounds, she has a greater likelihood of later developing Type 2 diabetes.

Likewise, women with polycystic ovary syndrome (PCOS) have an elevated risk. PCOS is a hormonal imbalance associated with insulin resistance and high levels of insulin in the blood—similar to the early stages of diabetes—that afflicts up to 10 percent of all women in their childbearing years.

It results in enlarged ovaries, irregular menstrual periods, failure to ovulate, weight gain, infertility and excessive body hair due to excessive testosterone levels. About 35 percent of women with PCOS go on to have diabetes and typically the disease progresses much more quickly than it does in women without PCOS.

In my practice, I have seen a low carbohydrate diet protocol will often lead to increased fertility.

The Danger of Inactivity

Although one can be overweight and still be physically active, inactivity is often a contributing factor to being overweight or obese. Exercise not only helps you maintain your healthy weight or weight loss, it also increases the ratio of muscle to fat in your body.

The more muscle mass you have, the higher your metabolism, which helps your burn more glucose and body fat. Also, importantly, the more muscle you have, the more responsive your body is to the effects of insulin.

In fact, a review of 14 studies has shown that even without significant weight loss, moderate exercise alone improves blood sugar control. Regular vigorous exercise works on multiple levels to reduce your risk for developing diabetes.

The Role of the Environment

A significant body of research links two toxins—arsenic and dioxins—to increased risk for diabetes.

Arsenic Assault

Although arsenic is present in the environment in many forms, the primary way in which the general public is exposed to this poison is through contaminated drinking water and pesticides.

People are also exposed to arsenic in medicines to treat conditions as diverse as psoriasis and leukemia, as well as in some wines (likely via arsenic-laced pesticides) and mineral waters. Individuals who work in certain occupations, such as processing metal ores, manufacturing glass and pharmaceuticals and producing or applying pesticides, are at heightened risk.

Several research studies have shown an association between exposure to arsenic and increased risk of developing diabetes.

Deadly Dioxin

The term dioxin includes a family of highly persistent fat-soluble compounds found most commonly in foods high on the food chain such as meat and dairy products. The most toxic form of dioxin is a byproduct of manufacturing and processing industries that use chlorine compounds.

These include paper pulp mills, water and waste processors and manufacturers of pesticides and polyvinyl chloride products. Dioxins also are spewed into the environment when chlorinated wastes are incinerated. In addition to a long list of health effects resulting from exposure to dioxins, high concentrations may alter glucose metabolism and hormonal levels.

Although the results of research have not been consistent, several findings suggest that dioxin exposure raises the risks for developing diabetes.

Research on men who were involved in aerial spraying of herbicides, including Agent Orange, were more likely to have diabetes, impaired glucose metabolism and impaired insulin production.

THE IMPORTANCE OF DIET

Talking about diabetes without discussing diet is like trying to put together a meal without any food. But I did want you to understand both the long progression to diabetes and other factors that influence whether this disease threatens your future before I get to the meat of the matter, so to speak.

First of all, let me repeat: You can prevent diabetes from ever developing by eating properly. Even if you already have disturbed blood sugar and insulin resistance, you can stop them in their tracks without drugs, simply by changing the way you eat.

This applies even if your parents and/or siblings have Type 2 diabetes.

The way of eating I advocate is not what the American Diabetic Association (ADA) recommends. Rather, instead of obsessing about fat and allowing plenty of sugar, white flour and other nutritionally deficient foods, as the ADA program does, my approach is derived from the work of Dr. Robert C. Atkins.

Although his low-carbohydrate diet is best known for its weight-loss results, eating only fiber- and nutrient-rich carbohydrates—and avoiding processed carbohydrates—in combination with a mix of protein sources and natural fats is ideally suited to managing blood sugar and insulin levels. At the same time, this way of eating makes it easy to keep weight under control—which is, of course, also key to avoiding diabetes.

In fact, at the time of his death, Dr. Atkins was at work on the book he felt was the culmination of this life's work. Atkins Diabetes Revolution: The Groundbreaking Approach to Preventing and Controlling Type 2 Diabetes (Morrow, 2004) was published posthumously.

Much of the book is based upon his observations working with thousands of patients, some of whom have since become my patients, who were able to correct their metabolic disorders by changing their diet, becoming physically active and following a supplement protocol similar to the one I will describe later in this chapter.

This book is, of course, about prevention, so my focus is on how carbohydrate control effectively prevents diabetes.

Why Low Fat Doesn't Work

Everyone agrees that keeping weight down reduces the risk of getting diabetes, as well as heart disease and a host of other conditions discussed in this book.

Long term, the best way to control your weight is to develop healthful eating habits and eat moderately. Do that, and unless you have a major metabolic disorder and are extremely inactive, you will arrive at a weight that is appropriate for your age and body type.

But if a diet—and I am speaking of a way of eating, not specifically a weight-loss diet—is impossible to maintain because it is lacking in flavor and leaves you hungry and with cravings for certain foods, it is only a matter of time before it becomes a former diet. In the decades since the American government has advocated a low-fat diet, the obesity epidemic has exploded.

Low Fat Is High Carb

A low-fat diet, by definition, is inherently a high carbohydrate diet. That's because when you restrict fat, you are restricting protein as well, since meat, poultry, fish, cheese, and most other forms of protein contain good amounts of fat.

What you are left with, then, is carbohydrates, which encompasses an array of foods. (Most foods contain some combination of fat, protein and carbohydrate.) Low-glycemic ("good") carbohydrates are typically whole foods like leafy green vegetables, brown rice, lentils, raspberries, and hundreds of other vegetables, fruits and whole grains.

Then there is the endless array of high-glycemic ("bad") carbohydrates that beckon from the supermarket shelves, including the processed, refined offerings such as cookies, chips, syrupy drinks, white bread and so on.

By definition, high glycemic foods have a dramatic impact on blood sugar levels within a couple of hours after consumption. In contrast, low glycemic foods raise blood sugar levels more slowly and moderately. In addition, dairy products contain carbohydrate along with fat and protein.

Carbs, Blood Sugar, and Insulin

While it is definitely possible to eat a high carbohydrate diet comprised primarily of fresh vegetables, whole grains and fruits—witness Mediterranean cuisine—with a modest amount of fish, cheese and meat, in this country, a so-called low-fat diet is usually packed with high-glycemic carbohydrates. And for someone with a genetic propensity to diabetes, that is a recipe for disaster. Here's why:

When you indulge in high-glycemic refined carbohydrate foods, your blood sugar quickly rises prompting your pancreas to release insulin to ferry the blood sugar to your cells. If you continue to eat this way, over time the cells become increasingly resistant to the effects of the insulin, stimulating the pancreas to produce even more insulin.

When the insulin finally does the trick, your blood sugar level dips so low that it can stimulate stress hormones that cause hunger and cravings for sweets and other carbohydrate foods. When you give into those cravings, the cycle repeats itself and the pounds pile on.

It is these cravings that distinguish the condition known as carbohydrate addiction, which makes it so difficult for some people to take control of their weight. In addition to the prompting the storage of excess glucose as body fat, the release of insulin has another dangerous result.

The fat is transported around your body in the bloodstream in the form of triglycerides. High triglycerides, you will recall, is an independent risk factor for diabetes.

Most Fats Are Fine

When you control carbohydrates, you don't have to keep track of how much fat—other than trans fats, known as hydrogenated or partially hydrogenated oils, which are to be avoided at all costs—you are eating.

That means that you can enjoy a lamb chop, salmon, olive oil on your vegetables and in your salad dressing and whipped cream on fresh raspberries, without feeling guilty. In fact, all these fats carry flavor, which makes food more satisfying.

When you eliminate most fat from your diet, you yearn for flavor, which can often lead to overeating. Fats provide a comforting satiety in a way that carbohydrates don't.

Dr. Salerno talks about Systemic yeast, also known as *Candida* and its relationship to weight loss

Amy came to my office by referral from another diet doctor. She had been on a low carb diet but her weight loss had stalled out and she was feeling depressed. Lately she had been craving sugar, but she associated this with a vacation to Mexico where everything had seemed to go South for her.

Her other symptoms included diarrhea, bloating, gas, fatigue, insomnia, and frequent lower abdominal pain, especially after eating. She had seen a succession of doctors, including a gastroenterologist, who told her she had irritable bowel syndrome (IBS) and recommended a high-fiber diet.

Like many women with similar problems, Amy had tried several regimens without success. She was really feeling bad. She had started out well in a weight loss program, but it had stalled out and she still had about 45 pounds to lose. But with the added problems of sugar cravings, fatigue, bloating, and pain, she had about given up.

I believed that Amy was suffering from systemic yeast, or *Candida*, often accompanied by dysbiosis which is an imbalance of the bacteria in the intestines secondary to parasites, yeast overgrowth, environmental or food sensitivities.

While I was taking her history, Amy reported she'd been on vacation in Mexico in the spring and that had been the end of success with her diet. I knew it was also probably the beginning of her problems with yeast and parasites.

We did a conventional work-up on her including a stool test which did, indeed, reveal the presence of parasites, systemic yeast, and imbalanced bacterial flora — the true underlying causes of her symptoms and the reason her diet was no longer working.

The parasites were the easy part. But the systemic yeast was the more difficult problem. But when she adhered to The Silver Cloud Diet, along with supplements, and some I.V. vitamins, we conquered her yeast and she lost the weight.

What is systemic yeast (*Candida*)?

Candida albicans is a fungal organism that is present in everyone's intestinal tract. It is normally kept under control by the immune system and by beneficial intestinal bacteria.

This balance is upset when these bacteria are destroyed (often by antibiotics), when our immune function is impaired (stress or illness), or when we develop environmental or food sensitivities.

Then, *Candida* begins to proliferate and invade and colonize our body tissues. It most commonly appears as a vaginal yeast infection or as oral thrush. But *Candida albicans* can also spread inside the body and become a systemic problem.

How does *Candida albicans* affect the body?

When *Candida* proliferates, it changes from its simple, relatively harmless form to an invasive form, with long root-like structures that penetrate the intestinal lining. Penetration can break down the boundary between the intestinal tract and the circulatory system.

This may allow introduction into the bloodstream of many substances which may be systemic allergens, poisons, or irritants. Partially digested proteins may enter the blood through the openings created by *Candida* (called leaky gut syndrome), which explains why individuals with *Candida* also often display a variety of food and environmental allergies.

What are some of the symptoms of *Candida* yeast infections?

While many of these symptoms may be caused by conditions other than candidiasis, a woman suffering from systemic yeast will typically experience a number of the following symptoms:

Weight gain: If she's been on a diet, it will no longer work. If she hasn't been on a diet, she may experience an unexplained weight gain.

Generalized: Fatigue, lethargy, migraine headaches, weakness, dizziness, sensory disturbances, hypoglycemia, muscle pain, respiratory problems, chemical sensitivities.

Gastrointestinal: Oral thrush, diarrhea, constipation, rectal itching, inflammatory bowel disease (IBD), flatulence, food sensitivities.

Genitourinary: Yeast vaginitis, menstrual and premenstrual problems, bladder inflammation, chronic urinary tract infections (UTI's), bladder inflammation, cystitis, PMS.

Dermatological: Eczema, acne, hives.

Mental and emotional: Panic attacks, confusion, irritability, memory loss, inability to concentrate, depression, insomnia, learning disability, short attention span.

Autoimmune: Multiple sclerosis, arthritis, systemic lupus erythematosus, myasthenia gravis, scleroderma, hemolytic anemia, sarcoidosis, thrombocytopenic purpura.

Diagnosis of systemic yeast (*Candida*) infection

A simple stool test can be done to determine if someone has *Candida* yeast overgrowth.

Treatment of systemic yeast (*Candida*) infection

We recommend dietary changes, supplements and lifestyle changes that provides a natural remedy for candidiasis.

Basic eating plan: The Silver Cloud Diet is a good basic diet to follow to rid yourself of a systemic yeast problem. Our diet is high in whole foods, with plenty of vegetables, protein, and natural fat, and virtually no simple sugars or processed carbohydrates.

Ideally the diet needs to be free of artificial colors, sweeteners and dyes.

1. *Avoid yeast-containing foods:*

- Beer, wine, and all other forms of alcohol
- Breads, rolls, pretzels, pastries, cookies, and sweet rolls
- B–complex vitamins and selenium products, unless labeled "yeast–free"
- Vinegar or foods containing vinegar, such as mustard, salad dressings, pickles, barbeque sauce, mayonnaise
- Commercially prepared foods such as soups, dry roasted nuts, potato chips, soy sauce, cider, natural root beer, olives, sauerkraut

2. *Avoid mold-containing and mold-supporting foods:*

- Pickled, smoked or dried meats, fish, and poultry
- Cured pork bacon
- All cheese, aged or fresh except cream cheese and fresh mozzarella
- Mushrooms
- Tempeh
- Soy sauce, tamari, and miso
- Peanuts, peanut products, and pistachios
- Herbs and teas that may be moldy
- Malt or foods containing malt
- Canned or prepared tomatoes (fresh tomatoes are fine)

3. *Avoid all sugars:*

- Honey, maple syrup, brown sugar
- Fruit juices (canned, bottled, or frozen)
- Dried fruits
- All processed sugar
- Anything containing high-fructose corn syrup
- High glycemic index foods

- All prepared and processed foods for a period of at least 4 weeks

What foods can you eat in a *Candida* **diet?**

- All fresh non-starchy vegetables — a large variety, raw, steamed, or sautéed in butter or olive oil with plenty of dark green leafy vegetables.
- Fresh protein at every meal, including beef, chicken, fish, turkey, eggs, and shellfish. Organic is best, but fresh is essential. Choose grass fed meats and wild caught fish.
- Unprocessed nuts and seeds, except peanuts.
- Unrefined cold-pressed olive, sesame, and coconut oils .
- Lemon juice with oil for salad dressing — this may be a prepared product, but be careful to avoid any salad dressing that contains vinegar.
- Beverages such as mineral or spring water, coffee, tea, and sugar-free cocktails
- Limited quantities of low-sugar fruit (three daily), unless you see a reaction, then limit to twice weekly. Avoid grapes, raisins, dates, prunes and figs..

How long does it take to **heal a systemic yeast infection?**

Most often, we recommend that you stay on this program for four months, then repeat the stool test. We usually find that enough progress has been made for a patient to wean off the antifungal agent and the probiotic supplement, and to moderate the anti-yeast diet at that point.

Where to go for **help with systemic yeast**

In our personal program, we provide pharmaceutical-grade supplements plus optional phone support from our Nurse–Educators. While the Personal Program isn't a medical practice, many women find the right combination of guidance and support from our nurses, who are highly trained. To learn more about the Program call The Salerno Center, **1-212-582-1700**.

Of course, you are always welcome to become a patient of The Salerno Center, located at 161 Madison Av, New York, New York. We have years of experience and great success in treating weight loss and other conditions including candida.

What's the Deal on Fluctuating Blood Sugars?

One of the most persistent problems that my patients tell me about when they come in for their first visit is a lack of energy, sometimes followed by explosive bursts of temper, foggy thinking, and other unpleasant effects from eating a diet high in sugars and carbohydrates.

Now, these people didn't come to me to correct their low energy, or quick temper, and often they don't even know there is a connection between the way they feel and what they eat. But the connection is clear. These patients are on a daily fun-house ride that seems painfully slow at times, then explosively fast at others.

In medicine, we know this to be the result of fluctuating blood sugars. You eat pancakes for breakfast with syrup, you feel like a million until about 10 am when all of a sudden you find yourself sweaty, cranky, irritable and sometimes even faint.

So what do you do? Grab a donut and a cup of coffee? I hope not, but that's often the answer. Then the fun house starts all over again, ultimately plunging you into a dark, scary place which feels like you'll never get out.

What most of these patients came to see me about is overweight and obesity. Many of them have tried punishing diets with almost no protein or fat, often vegetarian, and with such low calories that their body is thrown into a tantrum of fluctuating blood sugars.

The Dangers of Blood Sugar Fluctuation

A low level of blood sugar, referred to as hypoglycemia, results in an inadequate supply of glucose to the brain and leads to a considerable amount of malfunction.

Hypoglycemia can cause a number unpleasant symptoms including fatigue, weakness, dizziness, inability to concentrate, poor memory, anxiety, depression, irritability, heart palpitations and excessive sweating. It can even cause comas and seizures.

On the other end of the spectrum, a high level of blood sugar is referred to as hyperglycemia and is one of the key symptoms of diabetes. Hyperglycemia can cause similar symptoms to hypoglycemia such as fatigue, inability to concentrate, anxiety and depression.

However, it can also cause shortness of breath, nausea, dry mouth, and in severe cases, can even cause comas, nerve damage and blindness.

Blood sugar fluctuation puts a significant demand on the glands responsible for regulating it and this burden is one of the major reasons why fluctuating blood sugar is such a serious health concern. It's widely recognized as the cause of type 2 diabetes and is also associated with high blood pressure and heart disease.

How the Body Responds to Blood Sugar Fluctuation

High levels of blood sugar trigger the pancreas to respond in emergency like fashion by quickly releasing a large amount of insulin.

By facilitating the transport of blood glucose into cells and the conversion of excess blood glucose into body fat, the presence of insulin causes blood sugar to drop.

However, the large amount of insulin often causes too much glucose to be removed from the blood and results in a state of hypoglycemia.

The excessive drop in blood sugar creates another state of emergency and stimulates the adrenal glands to release cortisol. This increases blood sugar to a desirable level by facilitating the creation of glucose from body fat and muscle tissue, and also by stimulating the liver to create glucose from it's storage of glycogen.

While the mechanisms involved in blood sugar regulation provide us with an invaluable source of protection, they also put a significant physiological burden on the body.

The continuous demand put on the pancreas to produce excessive amounts of insulin is what eventually leads to type 2 diabetes. In similar fashion, the recurring need for the adrenal glands to produce cortisol can compromise their capacity as well and result in adrenal fatigue.

Although adrenal fatigue is not as widely recognized as diabetes, it can be equally problematic and result in susceptibility to significant health problems. Furthermore, any type of adrenal stimulation, including low blood sugar, invokes the universal stress response that is so frequently associated with poor health.

Tips for Regulating Blood Sugar

One of the best things you can do for your health is to keep your blood sugar at a relatively consistent level. The following tips will help to spare your body from the significant burden of blood sugar fluctuation and will help you maintain a steady mood and energy level while making your weight loss program both possible and pleasant.

• Choose The Silver Cloud Diet as your bible. This will give you a step-by-step instruction for regulating your blood sugars while you lose weight.

• Eliminate sugar and refined carbohydrates from your diet, or keep them to an absolute minimum. If you have any excess body fat, this will help you lose weight in addition to keeping your blood sugar stabilized.

• Minimize your intake of caffeine. Drink lemon water instead.

• Follow a consistent eating schedule, with 5 small meals a day and try not to go more than 4 hours without a meal.

• Some fruits and vegetables can cause blood sugar fluctuation just as easily as processed foods.

Bio-identical Hormone Replacement Therapy for Weight Loss Patients

Suzanne Somers and I met several years ago at a medical conference where we were both presenting. I admire her work getting the word out, and am grateful to her for including me in her list of *recommended doctors*, "I will personally send patients to see Dr. Salerno," says Ms. Somers.

Suzanne Somers has kindly included me in her books including ***Ageless, Breakthrough,*** and ***Knockout.***

My bio-identical hormone replacement (BHRT) therapy protocols are used not only in my New York practice, but also in practices I supervise in Japan and Brazil.

BHRT is key to anti-aging issues and is, in my experience, intertwined with weight issues in post menopausal women.

Not only Suzanne, but Oprah joins me in understanding the miraculous results that can obtain by designing a BHRT plan for each woman. Both Suzanne Somers and Oprah are enthusiastic users of BHRT, as is my co-author, Linda Eckhardt.

So what is Bio-identical Hormone Replacement Therapy exactly?

In a nutshell, BHRT, (bio-identical hormone replacement therapy) treats the symptoms of menopause, perimenopause and postmenopause.

Those symptoms can include hot flashes, bloating, weight gain, mood swings, and brain fog.

The Silver Cloud Diet is ideal for women because it focuses on high quality protein and natural fats, with plenty of fresh vegetables and fruits. We recommend supplements as well, but sometimes hormone imbalances must be addressed and that's when we turn to BHRT.

The first step we do is evaluate each woman's condition through an intake exam and complete blood work. Once we determine that a woman's natural hormones are in decline, either from menopause, or even hysterectomy, we begin a regimen of BHRT.

BHRT is not to be confused with synthetic hormone treatment, like the horse urine tabs that jolted a woman's body with enormous doses of estrogen and subjected her body to an increased risk for cancer of the breast and female organs.

The synthetics have been named in warnings by the FDA as dangerous to women's health and adding significant risk for female organ cancers.

On the contrary, BHRT are molecularly identical to endogenous hormones in the woman's body and are compounded for us in our own pharmacy.

We determine the exact mix for each woman and compound a blend of estrone, estradiol, and progesterone, as well as testosterone. (Yes, women need a bit of testosterone, too!)

In a case by case determination, we may add pregnenelone, dehydroepiandrosterone (DHEA) and estriol, which, to date are not approved for use in Canada or the U.S. but are widely used in Europe, Asia, and South America by us and many other medical practitioners. PREG helps mood and stabilizes hormones.

In addition to stabilizing a woman's moods, reducing or eliminating night sweats and hot flashes, the use of BHRT reduces the risk of osteoporosis and can be a real help to post menopausal women who are having trouble losing weight.

After putting a woman on a regimen of BHRT, we do periodic blood work and may adjust the dosage based on the results.

We find BHRT to be an enormous asset the clients on The Silver Cloud Diet who are in the age range, say 45 to 80, and we use it judiciously at the Salerno Centers worldwide.

Chronic Fatigue Syndrome – BHRT Diet and Nutrition

☐ *Can bio-identical hormones help chronic fatigue patients?*

By its very nature, chronic fatigue depletes the body's natural hormones. It's important to understand Chronic Fatigue as a self-cycling downward spiral that must be interrupted by a careful diagnosis then a regimen of bio-identical hormones, natural thyroid replacement, and a well-thought out all-natural diet of unprocessed foods as well as help optimizing sleep and rest.

In my practice I often find chronic fatigue patients deficient in hormones. Replacing them as naturally as possible is the best way to balance the body so the patient can quickly experience symptom relief. These hormones include estrogen, progesterone, testosterone, DHEA and pregnenolone.

☐ *What role do bio-identical hormone treatments play in fatigued patients?*

Balancing the hormone deficiency with Bio-Identical Hormones when combined with diet and support will increase strength, stamina, mood and motivation. We run a comprehensive blood test to determine the exact combination of bio-identical hormones that will best balance each patient's body.

Thyroid health is also an important factor. We do a special test to get a more in-depth view of how the patient's thyroid is working.

This test is called the Thyroid Releasing Hormone Stimulation Test (TRH). The TRH test is different from the more common TSH test and sometimes catches imbalances that the TSH test cannot.

Making sure the thyroid is functioning properly is essential for total wellness and relief from fatigue. I prescribe a natural thyroid replacement which is much more effective than the synthetic treatment often suggested.

☐ *What role do diet and nutrition play in CFS?*

A well-balanced diet of organic, unprocessed foods with sufficient protein and natural fats is most beneficial to the Chronic Fatigue patient.

A poor diet is one of the most important factors that contribute to fatigue. This life changing plan is beneficial to the CFS patient as well as to people who wish to normalize their weight, increase their stamina and general health to look forward to a long and vigorous life.

I have had great success with CFS patients by combining The Silver Cloud Diet with a regimen of bio-identical hormones, thyroid, and recommendations for improved sleep and exercise.

☐ *In very basic terms, how can you change your diet to improve CFS symptoms?*

I highly recommend a low carb diet of unprocessed and organic foods to improve CFS symptoms. The diet MUST consist of organic food as much as possible and very few or no refined carbohydrates or processed foods.

☐ *What specific foods (or food groups) should you focus on, and in what amounts?*

Focus on wild caught fish, organic vegetables, grass-fed meats, organic eggs and full-fat cheeses which are all well tolerated by the CFS patient. Add dark colored fruits including berries which are also recommended.

☐ *What foods should you try to avoid? How can these worsen CFS symptoms?*

I love this question. It's so easy and yet so hard for most Americans to realize how important it is to eliminate all processed foods, sugars and bad carbs such as highly refined carbohydrates in store-bought breads, cookies, chips, crackers and other snack foods that are packaged or boxed.

Eating whole, unprocessed organic foods helps the body's natural functions to be optimized, excess weight is lost and overall health is restored. I am not only recommending a special diet for the CFS patient, but a plan to improve the health of every member of the family.

☐   *Is it a good idea to use caffeine to try to alleviate CFS symptoms? Why or why not?*

Caffeine in moderation, generally, is acceptable as it can increase energy.

☐   *What role does caffeine play in regard to CFS?*

Overuse of caffeine or any stimulant including sugar and all its derivatives can make it difficult to fall asleep and stay asleep. Getting plenty of rest is imperative in allowing the body to heal and to stay in balance. No coffee or caffeine-laced products (including chocolate) after the afternoon.

☐   *What about ADHD drugs? What are your thoughts on these in regard to CFS?*

Stimulants and ADHD drugs must be avoided as they will cause long term issues and eventually serious side effects which can, if untreated, be fatal. Some good alternatives to these stimulants are all-natural supplements that can replace what is most deficient in the body. Supplements such as L-Carnatine, CoQ10, D-Ribose, B12, and L-Taurine work very nicely and have no side effects.

At www.thesilverclouddiet.com, we offer healthy all natural supplements to help the CFS patient as well as those who wish to lose weight. Order from us for prompt delivery.

THE IMPORTANCE OF SUPPLEMENTS

A good supplement program acts as an insurance policy, even when you follow a healthful diet. The following supplements promote the metabolism of carbohydrates, improve insulin sensitivity, lower triglycerides and act as anti-inflammatories.

Our office patients may elect to receive supplements by weekly IV infusions. We also prescribe pure, organic supplements and compounds made especially for our patients and for our website readers (www.thesilverclouddiet.com).

Biotin

A water-soluble B vitamin, also known as vitamin H, biotin is key to the metabolism of energy, enabling four essential enzymes to break down carbohydrates into glucose, fats into fatty acids and protein into amino acids.

Produced in the body by certain types of intestinal bacteria, biotin is also found in foods such as brewer's yeast, nutritional yeast, oat bran, whole grains, nuts and nut butters, egg yolks, sardines, legumes, liver and other organ meats, bananas, cauliflower and mushrooms.

People with Type 2 diabetes often are deficient in biotin. Long-term use of antibiotics can also depress levels.

Optimal daily dose: 2-4 mg per day. Note: Biotin appears to work synergistically with chromium to control blood sugar, so be sure to take the two supplements together.

Chromium

Like biotin, the trace mineral chromium plays a role in the metabolism of carbohydrates, protein and fat, helping your body metabolize fat, turn protein into muscle and convert carbohydrate into energy. Chronium used to abundant in the soil, but industrial farming and the overuse of pesticides and herbicides have leached the soils of most of this vital nutrient.

Chromium is necessary to make glucose tolerance factor, which enhances the action of insulin, facilitating the process by which glucose is transported to the liver, muscle and fat cells, where it can be converted for energy as needed, thereby keeping blood sugar levels under control.

Deficiency in chromium results in impaired glucose tolerance, insulin resistance and diabetes-like symptoms. In addition, chromium acts as an appetite suppressant.

Chromium supplements have also been shown to improve glucose tolerance and reduce abnormally high blood levels of insulin in pregnant women with gestational diabetes. Since heart disease is often a complication of diabetes, improvements in cholesterol and triglycerides are valuable benefits.

Vigorous exercise can deplete the body's stores of chromium. Processing foods also depletes them of most of the trace mineral Trace amounts of chromium are found in many foods, among them brewers yeast, beef, cheese, leafy dark greens, mushrooms, shellfish and barley.

Optimal daily dose: 200-600 mcg per day. Note: Chromium should be taken with biotin for maximum effectiveness.

Vanadium

Along with biotin and chromium, vanadium helps get the proper amounts of glucose into the body's cells. This trace mineral is found in black pepper, mushrooms, sunflower and safflower seeds and oil, olive oil, shellfish, parsley, dill seed, buckwheat, oats, rice, green beans, carrots, cabbage, radishes and eggs. In vivo and in vitro studies have shown this that vanadium mimics the effects of insulin.

Vanadium can lower blood sugar levels and improve sensitivity to insulin in both Type 1 and Type 2 diabetes.

In parts of the world where industrial farming practices have not leached the soils of vanadium and selenium, there are lower than average rates of heart disease. Nonetheless, too much vanadium can be dangerous.

Optimal daily dose: 30-60 mg vanadyl sulfate or 1-2 mg vanadyl per day. Note: Excessive levels of vanadyl can be toxic so take care not to exceed dosage.

Coenzyme Q-10

This micronutrient is produced by the body but production slows with age. Coenzyme Q-10 plays an important role in producing energy for the mitochondria found in every cell in your body. People with diabetes typically have lower levels of Co-Q-10 than healthy people.

Optimal daily dose: 100-300 mg per day.

Alpha Lipoic Acid

The antioxidant alpha lipoic acid assists the body in using glucose, which enables it to improve blood sugar control. In one study, people with Type 2 diabetes who were give intravenous supplemental alpha lipoic acid (ALA) saw an increase in insulin release and a reduction in blood sugar levels.

One way in which antioxidants, of which ALA is one, help fight diabetes is by neutralizing free radicals in your body involved in the development of insulin resistance. Supplementing with ALA has been shown to enhance uptake of glucose by tissues.

One serious complication of diabetes is nerve damage called diabetic neuropathy, which results in pain, tingling and numbness in the extremities. It can be relieved with supplemental ALA. One study showed that nerve function was restored after four months on high oral doses. " Alpha Lipoic acid improves nerve blood flow, reduces oxidative stress and improves distal nerve conduction in experimental diabetic neuropathy."

Optimal daily dose: 600-1000 mg per day.

N-Acetyl-L-Cysteine

N-acetyl cysteine (NAC) is a form of the amino acid cysteine, which helps the body synthesize the antioxidant glutathione that has been shown to improve insulin sensitivity. When insulin levels are high, free radicals flourish, which can destroy various types of tissue.

Optimal daily dose: 600-1200 mgs per day. Note: NAC should be accompanied by 15 mg of zinc and 2 mg of copper per day.

Gymnema Sylvestre

Also known as Gurmar and Meshashringi, the leaves of the plant gymnema sylvestre have been used for centuries in Ayuvedic medicine to regulate glucose metabolism. In fact, the Hindi name gurmar translates as "sugar destroyer."

Unlike a prescription drug, gymnema lowers blood sugar levels gradually by helping regenerate the beta cells in the pancreas that secrete insulin, thus raising insulin levels. (Unlike insulin and other drugs, gymnema won't reduce blood sugar to dangerous levels).

It also interferes with glucose absorption in the intestine, which helps keep the pancreas from releasing too much insulin. The herb also helps the uptake of glucose by the cells and keeps adrenaline from stimulating the liver to produce glucose.

Finally, it banishes the taste of sugar, which suppresses cravings for sweets, making it easier to lose weight.

Optimal daily dose: 500 mcg. per day

Banaba Leaf Extract

Long used in the Philippines as a natural plant insulin for blood sugar control, banaba leaf appears to balance blood sugar by promoting healthy insulin levels and stimulating the transport of glucose into cells. It also is said to help control cravings, particularly for carbohydrates and may promote weight loss.

In a clinical study of people with Type 2 diabetes who received a standardized extract of banaba leaf that contained 1-percent corosolic acids showed a 30 percent decrease in blood sugar levels after two weeks.

Optimal daily dose: 50 mg per day.

Cinnamon Bark

Next time you sprinkle cinnamon on your cappuccino or your oatmeal, you may also be cutting your risk for diabetes and cardiovascular disease.

The familiar spice is a potent antioxidant with the potential to help maintain healthy blood sugar and cholesterol levels. The Chinese used cinnamon for an array of medical complaints ranging from diarrhea to influenza as long as 4,000 years ago.

It was also used, as many spices were, to preserve food in the days before refrigeration.

Regular supplementation with cinnamon may be able to reduce fasting blood sugar, triglycerides, LDL cholesterol and total cholesterol. Supplementation does not improve glycemic control in postmenopausal women.

Optimal daily dose: 125-250 mg per day.

Magnesium

Magnesium lowers blood glucose levels, increases insulin sensitivity, and calms the sympathetic nervous system.

Although the relationship between magnesium and diabetes has been studied for decades, it is still poorly understood. However, what is known about diabetes and magnesium embodies a persuasive list encouraging supplementation:

Low magnesium levels are common findings in non-insulin-dependent diabetic patients (Paolisso et al. 1989). In fact, diabetes is a frequent cause of secondary hypomagnesemia (lower blood levels of magnesium). Poorly controlled diabetics excrete more magnesium than do non-diabetics.

Magnesium assists in the maintenance of functional beta cells (insulin factories) (Kowluru et al. 2001). Scientists believe that a magnesium deficiency interrupts insulin secretion and its activity. Magnesium, by enhancing the action of insulin, improves insulin's ability to transport glucose into the cell.

Magnesium increases the number and sensitivity of insulin receptors (Waterfall 2000).

An increase in red blood cell magnesium significantly and positively correlated with an increase in both insulin secretion and action. Correction of low erythrocyte magnesium concentrations may allow for improved glucose handling, particularly in elderly diabetic patients (Paolisso et al. 1992, 1993a).

As magnesium levels plummet, the incidence of diabetic complications escalates.

Magnesium is the mineral of choice to reduce hyper-responsiveness occurring in the sympathetic nervous system (SNS). This is important to the diabetic because when the SNS is alerted, blood glucose levels tend to be higher.

The SNS is also associated with fostering greater levels of stress and anxiety, earning its reputation as the "flight or fight" division. Since diabetes is considered to be a disease promulgated by stress, supplementation that favors an inner calm is of significant advantage.

Optimal daily dose: 750 mg. daily, divided into 2 doses

Resveratrol

Neuroprotective effects: In November 2008, researchers at the Weill Medical College of Cornell University reported that dietary supplementation with resveratrol significantly reduced plaque formation in animal brains, a component of Alzheimer's and other Neurodegenerative diseases.

In humans it is theorized that oral doses of resveratrol may reduce beta amyloid plaque associated with aging changes in the brain. Researchers theorize that one mechanism for plaque eradication is the ability of resveratrol to chelate (bind) copper. The neuroprotective effects have been confirmed in several animal model studies.

The anti-inflammatory effects of resveratrol have been demonstrated in several animal model studies. Resveratrol has showed promise as a potential therapy for arthritis.

Cardioprotective effects: It has long been known that moderate drinking of red wine reduces the risk of heart disease. This is best known as "the French paradox."

Studies suggest that resveratrol in red wine may play an important role in this phenomenon. The cardioprotective effects of resveratrol are also theorized to be a form of preconditioning—the best method of cardioprotection, rather than direct therapy.

Anti-diabetic effects: Resveratrol ameliorates common diabetes symptoms, such as polyphagia, polydipsia, and body weight loss. In human clinical trials, resveratrol has lowered blood sugar levels in both Phase Ib and Phase IIa.

Antiviral effects: Studies show that resveratrol inhibits herpes simplex virus (HSV) types 1 and 2 replication by inhibition of an early step in the virus replication cycle.

Studies also show that resveratrol inhibit varicella-zoster virus, certain influenza virus, respiratory viruses, and human cytomegalovirus. Furthermore, resveratrol synergistically enhances the anti-HIV-1 activity of several anti-HIV drugs.

Optimal daily dose: 500 mgs

Part II:

How to Start The Silver Cloud Diet

The Silver Cloud Detox: The Full Fat Fast gives your body a rest from the assaults of the Western Diet. Getting rid of carbs from your diet will quickly put your body into fat-burning mode, and if you adhere to this for two weeks you will lose from five to fifteen pounds and two inches off your waist.

Put this up on your refrigerator for ready reference.

Here's a step-by-step guide to your day on the **Silver Cloud Detox:** *The Full Fat Fast*:

- Within one hour of rising each morning, eat two large organic eggs, cooked any way you like (suggestions and recipes below). You can add a side of bacon or sausage or ham if you want, and you can also have coffee or tea with cream and sweetener.

- Three hours later have a small snack: a stick of string cheese, a handful of nuts, jerky, an ounce of sausage, or even some pork skins. Add another cup of coffee or tea with cream and sweetener if you wish.

- Eat lunch three hours later: two ounces of cooked steak, hamburger, lamb chop, pork chop, any preservative free sausage, salmon, sardines with mustard, tuna salad made with regular mayonnaise. You may even choose a couple more eggs, perhaps made into a salad.

- Three hours later have another snack of about fifteen nuts (macadamias, brazils, walnuts, hazelnuts, pecans, or pistachios are fine). A hand full of pork skins, a stick of cheese, or some jerky is also ok.

- Have your dinner three hours later: another two ounces of steak, burger, chops, poultry or fish.

- Drink lots of water-based liquids during the day, at least 64 ounces. Coffee with heavy cream is fine, iced tea with fresh mint, or lemon water, which is ice water with a squirt of lemon juice and a packet of sugar substitute. Stevia is best, but sucralose (Splenda) is fine too.

- Remember that these products are much sweeter than sugar, so use a small amount in the water. Plain, old fashioned water is perhaps the best choice. Just drink and drink and drink.

- On the first day of your fast, measure yourself. Weigh in and write it down. Use a tape measure around your waist. After a week, weigh yourself again, and then weigh yourself one more time at the end of the *Full Fat Fast* one week later.

- After three or four days, you may experience constipation. Correct with a daily serving of Miracle Noodles (www.miraclenoodle.com) OR (shirataki at the Asian market nearest you.) These all-fiber, no carb, no calorie foods from Asia are a life saver.

- See recipes at the miracle noodle site, or simply do what we do, rinse the noodles in boiling water, drain, put up in zip locks, then long about mid afternoon, eat three tablespoons or so with a drop or two of your favorite no-carb salad dressing. You will never be hungry, you will never be constipated. This works.

FOODS TO ADORE	
Fats	extra virgin olive oil, butter, unrefined flax oil, fresh lard, foie gras, nuts (walnuts, pecans, brazil nuts, and hazelnuts)
Proteins	organic or grass fed beef, pork, veal, lamb, game, chicken, turkey, duck and other fowl (where possible). Chicken or veal liver, nitrate free bacon and sausage, all seafood from cold, deep water (including codfish, halibut, and salmon), shellfish, and eggs
Dairy	butter, raw milk cheeses, organic full fat milk, yogurt, buttermilk, heavy and sour cream from pasture-fed cows
Beverages	water, lemon water, coffee, tea (at least 64 ounces a day)
Condiments	sea salt, best quality balsamic vinegar, apple cider vinegar, rice wine vinegar, mayonnaise, mustards, soy sauce, fish sauce

FOODS TO ABHOR	
Fats	highly processed vegetable oils like canola or soybean, margarine, vegetable shortening
Proteins	processed meats
Dairy	processed cheeses, reduced or non-fat dairy products
Carbohydrates	For the detox phase, avoid starchy fruits and vegetables, any highly processed carbohydrate, white flour or anything made from white flour (including bread, cookies, crackers, pastas, and dry cereals), high fructose corn syrups, refined sugars, irradiated or genetically modified grains, chocolate mixed with sugar in any form
Beverages	Soda, including "diet" or "sugar free", full strength fruit juices, beer, wine, rice milk, soy milk
Condiments	catsup, commercial baking powder, MSG, artificial flavors, additives and colors

Eggs, your new best friend

Eggs contain the highest quality source of protein available and almost every essential vitamin and mineral needed by humans, which is why in the *Full Fat Fast* you'll be eating two every morning for breakfast. In fact, egg protein is of such high quality that it is used as the standard by which other proteins are compared.

Eggs have a biological value (efficacy with which protein is used for growth) of 93.7%. Comparable values are 84.5% for milk, 76% for fish, and 74.3% for beef. Eggs really are the best protein money can buy, and it has all those other valuable vitamins and minerals too.

Nutrient (unit)	Large Organic Whole Egg	Egg White	Egg Yolk
Calories (kcal)	72	17	55
Protein (g)	6.29	3.60	2.70
Carbohydrate (g)	0.39	0.21	0.61
Total Fat (g)	4.97	0.06	4.51
Saturated fat (g)	1.55	0	1.624
Monosaturated fat (g)	1.905	0	1.995
Polysaturated fat (g)	0.682	0	0.715
Cholesterol (mg)	212	0	210
Thiamin (mg)	0.035	0.001	0.03
Riboflavin (mg)	0.239	0.145	0.09
Folate (mcg)	24	1	25
Vitamin B6 (mg)	0.071	0.002	0.059
Vitamin B12 (mcg)	0.65	0.03	0.33
Vitamin A (IU)	244	0	245
Vitamin E (mg)	0.48	0	0.44
Vitamin D (IU)	18	0	18
Choline (mg)	125.6	-	-
Calcium (mg)	26	2	22
Iron (mg)	0.92	0.03	0.46
Magnesium (mg)	6	4	1
Copper (mg)	0.05	0.01	0.01
Zinc (mg)	0.56	0.01	0.39
Sodium (mg)	70	55	8
Potassium (mg)	67	54	19
Phosphorus (mg)	96	5	66
Lutein & Zeaxanthin	166	0	186

(mcg)			

Nutritional Content of a Large Egg

Source: USDA National Nutrient Database

Eggs have long been an important contributor to the nutritional quality of the American diet. According to the USDA, eggs supply a higher percentage of nutrients to the diet than calories. While eggs provide only 1.3% of the average caloric intake, they contain 6% of the recommended dietary allowance (RDA) for riboflavin, 5% of the folate, 4% of the vitamin E and vitamin A, and almost 4% of the protein.

Nutrient		Percentage (%)
	Food Energy	1.3
	Protein	3.9
	Fat	2.0
	Vitamin A	4.3
	Vitamin E	4.3
	Riboflavin	6.4
	Vitamin B6	2.1
	Vitamin B12	3.7
	Folate	5.1
	Iron	2.4
	Phosphorous	3.6
	Zinc	2.8

We're sure you might have heard though that eggs are linked to heart disease. This is a myth – thirty years has scientific research have yet to link the two. In fact, a study completed in 2007 shows that while eggs don't increase the chance of heart disease in healthy adults, they may be associated with a decrease in blood pressure (besides having tremendous nutritional value).

Eggs a dozen ways

Chefs have long considered the mastery of egg cookery to be an excellent way to measure incoming chefs. Master French Chef Fernana Point (1897-1955) would test visiting chefs with a challenge to show him how they fried a simple egg, declaring that the easiest dishes were often the most difficult to prepare. When, inevitably, the new chef insulted the egg with the sizzling hot surface of a frying pan, Point would cry, "Stop, unhappy man - you are making a dog's bed of it!"

Soft Boiled Eggs

For each person, place two large eggs in a small bowl of warm tap water to cover. Fill a small saucepan three quarter full of water. Raise to a boil and then add a pinch of salt. Lower the eggs in a spoon into gently boiling water. Cook 4 minutes for a soft center and 6 minutes for medium. Lift eggs out with a spoon, run under cold tap water a moment, then transfer to an egg cup. Nip the end of the egg off with a knife and dive in.

Hard Boiled Eggs

Follow directions above but cook the eggs for 10 minutes. You can also place eggs in the pan of water to begin. Once the eggs are cooked, plunge them into cold water. Once they're cooled, crack and shell them, and now you're ready for devilled eggs, egg salad, or endless garnishes and nutritional boosts to salads.

Poached Eggs

The beauty of poached eggs is that you can cook as many as 15 at a time if you're having a party or you can just cook yourself a couple. The key is to use the freshest possible eggs so they'll hold their shape. In at least four inches of simmering water with a tablespoon of vinegar, gently slip the eggs into the water and watch until the white has set up and the yolk looks firm. Use a slotted spoon to lift them from the water. Hold a towel in your other hand, and let the excess water drip off, then slide the egg in to a bowl.

Coddled Eggs

No, these eggs haven't been hugged and kissed, but rather are eggs that are cooked in these cute little porcelain dishes available at any cooking supply store. Brush the dish with butter, break the eggs in, screw on the metal top, and lower into barely boiling water. Cook 7 to 8 minutes, then lift out of the water. Use tongs, don't lift through the ring on the top. Place the porcelain coddlers on a plate and serve. The thing that gets coddled is the person who gets to eat them. Makes you feel so special.

It's what the French call Oeufs en Cocotte, or eggs baked in a dish. Simply use any small baking dish, slather it with butter, break a couple eggs in, season with salt and pepper, add a splash of cream on top, and place it in a 325 degree oven for about 12 to 14 minutes. Transfer the dish to a plate and serve. I think of this kind of egg cookery as a lot of sizzle for the simple egg.

Microwaved Eggs

You shouldn't try cooking eggs in the shells in the microwave unless you're interested in science experiments regarding the difficulty of removing cooked egg from the walls of the oven. They will explode. However, you can make quick and easy scrambled eggs.

Place two eggs in a well-buttered 10 ounce custard cup. Season to taste with salt and pepper. Add 1 tablespoon cream and whisk with a fork. Cook uncovered from 1 to 2 minutes, whisking once in the middle, but just until liquid egg is no longer visible.

Then remove from the oven and cover and let stand for a minute or so. Now that's a pretty quick meal eh? Three minutes tops.

Fried Eggs

Now this is all about the pan, a fresh egg, some butter, and the correct temperature. You've probably been served eggs that had a whiff of burnt hair and crispy icky edges. That was a result of a too-hot pan.

But frying eggs should be simple. Preheat a perfectly clean heavy skillet over medium heat. Then add butter and swirl to melt it. Break eggs into the pan, reduce heat to low, add a teaspoon of water, cover and wait a minute. Open up the lid. The eggs should be just about cooked, whites set, yolk looking shiny. Transfer to a plate, season with salt and pepper and eat.

Scrambled Eggs

Choose an 8 to 10 inch heavy skillet. Preheat over medium heat. Meanwhile whisk a couple eggs with a teaspoon of water and salt and pepper. Add a knob of butter to the pan and swirl to melt it. Pour in the eggs, and reduce heat to low. Cook, stirring from time to time, until the eggs look a bit like runny cottage cheese.

Take care not to overcook or you'll have a bad version of yellow rubber boots that smell something like burning hair. The eggs should clump up when you run the spatula under them and once you see there's no more wet egg, quickly transfer them to your warmed breakfast plate.

Pickled Eggs

Hemingway considered the pickled eggs on the bar in one of his famous short stories. Nothing could be simpler to make. Hard cook a dozen eggs. Shell them and place them in a half gallon jar. Pour the pickling mixture over them, cover and refrigerate. Then when you need a quick pick-me- up, eat yourself a pickle.

1 quart vinegar (malt or cider) *
2 tablespoons freshly grated ginger
1 tablespoon black peppercorns
1 teaspoon allspice or pickling spice

Combine ingredients in a saucepan with 1 cup water and raise to a rolling boil. Transfer to a large jar. Add boiled and peeled eggs. Cover and refrigerate, at least 24 hours but up to 1 month.

*remember to avoid vinegar if you have a yeast problem.

Perfect Omelets

Get yourself a nice, new 8 to 12-inch omelet pan (a very clean nonstick pan will also suffice, but do not use Teflon). Which size pan you use depends upon your particular view of the omelet. If you're of the "You can't be too rich or too thin" school, choose the larger pan.

If you prefer your omelet fluffy and a little thicker, choose the smaller. Purists will tell you the omelet should have NO browning but should simply be golden yellow. Personally, I like a little color on my omelet, not only for the look of it, but because the browning also complicates the flavor.

Next, prepare the filling. If you're grating cheese, use a microplane and grate it right onto the dinner plate you will ultimately use. Then, preheat the skillet over medium low heat.

Whisk 2 eggs with salt and pepper and a teaspoon of water. Melt a knob of butter in the skillet, swirling to cover every inch. Pour the eggs into the skillet. Let them set without touching for a minute, then begin lifting the skillet on one side and then the other so the runny part in the middle can move to the side.

Pick up an edge and see if it is beginning to color up. Add grated cheese to half of it, use your spatula to fold it over itself to turn it in half and remove to the plate. Now what could be simpler? All of this is done in under 5 minutes.

Deviled Eggs

6 large eggs
½ teaspoon white wine vinegar*
1 tablespoon sour cream
1 tablespoon mayonnaise
1 tablespoon minced shallot
2 teaspoons capers, finely minced
Salt and pepper and a dash of cayenne pepper
1 tablespoon minced fresh chives or dill

To hard-cook eggs, bring pan of water to simmer. Gently lay eggs in the water, return to simmer and cook for 8 minutes. Drain and cool eggs in ice water just until cool enough to handle. Peel eggs and chill again in ice water until cooled. (This keeps yolks perfectly yellow, and the shell slips off easily when the eggs are slight warm.) Slice eggs in half lengthwise and remove yolks. Mash yolks with vinegar, sour cream, mayonnaise, shallot, capers, salt and pepper to taste, cayenne pepper, and chives or dill. Add a dollop to each cooked egg white.

*remember to avoid vinegar if you have a yeast problem.

Egg Salad

1/2 dozen large eggs, hard cooked and peeled
½ cup mayonnaise
½ teaspoon curry powder
1 teaspoon pickle relish
1 teaspoon minced onion
Salt and pepper to taste

Chop eggs into a bowl. Mix with mayo, curry, pickle relish, onion and salt and pepper to taste. Place in a bowl and cover. Refrigerate up to a week.

Other Silver Cloud Detox: *Full Fat Fast* Recipes

We don't offer too many recipes for the detox phase. The simplest thing to do is go to a great butcher and fish monger, look in the case and buy yourself grass-fed meats and wild-caught fish and shell fish.

At home, cook them in a pan with butter and/or olive oil, seasoned with a simple sprinkling of sea salt and cracked black pepper.

You'll have sumptuous dinners in under 10 minutes, no matter what you choose and, because you've chosen high quality foods to begin with, it will be simple to stay on the plan and eat well.

Saucy Vodka Chicken

This spicy, smoky chicken is perfect whether you're cooking for yourself for weeknight dinners or for an impromptu party. Start with three chickens, whole or broken up into parts. If you bought whole chickens, you'll have leftover backs for stock.

We think of these brightly flavored chicken pieces as the perfect Tupperware lunch item. And don't worry about that vodka. Since it has no carbs, it's perfectly all right to use.

Makes 12 to 16 servings.

1 cup soy sauce
1/2 cup vodka
3 packets sugar substitute (or to taste)
½ cup extra virgin olive oil, divided
6 large cloves garlic, smashed
4 tablespoons Asian sesame oil
3 tablespoons ground cumin
1 teaspoon dried hot red-pepper flakes (or to taste)
6 chicken wings (2 lb total)
6 chicken breasts cut in half with skin and bones (4 lb total)
6 chicken thigh-drumstick (3 lb total)
1/2 lime, juice + grated zest
Accompaniment: lime wedges

Stir together soy sauce, vodka, sugar substitute, oil, garlic, sesame oil, cumin, and red-pepper flakes in a large glass measure. Divide chicken pieces among large sealable bags, then divide marinade among bags and seal, pressing out excess air. Put bags in a large bowl (in case of leaks) and marinate the chicken, chilled, 2 hours to overnight.

Put oven racks in upper and lower thirds of oven and preheat oven to 450°F. Brush 2 large shallow baking pans with oil. Divide chicken between pans, skin side down. Pour marinade into a 4-quart wide saucepan. Roast chicken in oven 12 minutes. Turn chicken over and switch the pans and continue to until cooked through and lightly browned, 13 to 18 minutes more.

Transfer chicken to platter. While chicken roasts, gently boil marinade until reduced to about 1 1/2 cups, 20 to 25 minutes. Drizzle chicken with some of sauce and serve remainder on the side. Squeeze juice from lime half all over chicken before serving.

Leftover sauce keeps in an airtight container, chilled, up to 3 days. Cool completely, uncovered, then chill, covered. Bring to room temperature before using.

Nutritional readout: 460 calories, FAT 34 g., Protein 35.6 g., carb 7.2 g, fiber 1.2 g.

Sautéed Flank Steak with an Anchovy Sauce

Here's French cooking 101. A simple steak cooked and fanned out onto the plate in a mouthwatering presentation. If you prefer another cut, feel free to substitute. Anything from a skirt to a filet mignon works well.

Makes 4 servings.

1 flank steak, about 16 ounces
Juice and grated zest of 1 lime
Kosher salt and cracked black pepper to taste
Whiff cayenne pepper
2 tablespoons extra virgin olive oil
1 2-oz. can anchovies in oil (reserve oil)
6 large cloves garlic, smashed
1 green onion and top, minced
½ cup water

Rub steak with 1 tablespoon lime juice and sprinkle with salt and pepper 10 minutes before cooking. Heat olive oil and oil from canned anchovies in large, heavy skillet over high heat. When hot, add steak and cook about 2 minutes on each side for medium rare, or to preferred doneness. When steak is cooked, transfer to a warmed plate to rest a few minutes.

Meanwhile, crush anchovy fillets with chopped garlic. Add to green onion in the pan drippings and cook about 30 seconds. Add water and boil 30 seconds, wiping up bits from the bottom of the pan. Swirl butter into the pan to melt. Pour over steak, sprinkle with more lime juice, and cut into thin slices and serve on warmed plates.

Nutritional Readout: 265 calories, FAT 15.3., PROTEIN 28.5., CARB 1.9 g., FIBER .02

Bourbon Chicken Liver Paté

We Love Three Little Pigs brand of patés, http://www.3pigs.com/,but if you'd like to create your own luxury on a diet. Make a pan of this pate, refrigerate it and eat a 2 ounce slice every three hours.

Makes 8 to 10 servings.

1 1/2 sticks (3/4 cup) unsalted butter
1 cup finely chopped onion
1 large garlic clove, minced
1 teaspoon minced fresh thyme or 1/4 teaspoon dried
1 teaspoon minced fresh marjoram or 1/4 teaspoon dried
1 teaspoon minced fresh sage or 1/4 teaspoon dried
sea salt and black pepper to taste
1/8 teaspoon ground allspice
1 lb chicken livers
2 tablespoons bourbon

Special equipment: a 2 1/2-cup crock or terrine or several small ramekins

Garnish: a fresh thyme, marjoram, or sage sprig

Melt 1 stick butter in a large nonstick skillet over moderately low heat, and then cook onion and garlic, stirring, until softened, about 5 minutes. Add herbs, salt, pepper, allspice, and livers and cook, stirring; until livers are cooked outside but still pink when cut open, about 8 minutes.

Stir in bourbon and remove from heat. Purée mixture in a food processor until smooth, then transfer pâté to crock and smooth top.

Melt remaining 1/2 stick butter in a very small heavy saucepan over low heat, then remove pan from heat and let butter stand 3 minutes. If using herb garnish, put sprig on top of pâté. Skim froth from butter, then spoon enough clarified butter over pâté to cover its surface, leaving milky solids in bottom of pan.

Chill pâté until butter is firm, about 30 minutes, then cover with plastic wrap and chill at least 2 hours more.

Nutritional readout: 187 calories, FAT 16.g, PROTEIN 8.g., CARB 1.5., FIBER .4 g

Apple-Smoked Pork Loin

Pork loin is an easy meat to cook and keep on hand in the refrigerator for quick lunches during the week.

Makes 8 servings

3 cups apple wood or orange wood chips or 6 to 8 apple wood or orange wood chunks
1 2- to 2-1/2-pound boneless pork top loin roast (single loin)
2 teaspoons dried oregano, crushed
4 cloves garlic, minced
1/2 teaspoon sea salt and freshly milled black pepper OR to taste

At least 1 hour before cooking, soak wood chips or chunks in enough water to cover. Meanwhile, trim fat from roast. Place roast in a shallow dish. In a small bowl, stir together dried oregano, garlic, salt, and pepper. Sprinkle evenly over all sides of roast; rub in with your fingers.

Drain wood chips. Prepare grill for indirect grilling. Test for medium-low heat above drip pan. Sprinkle half of the drained wood chips over the coals.

Place roast on grill rack directly over drip pan. Cover and grill for 1 to 1 1/2 hours or until internal temperature registers 155° degree F on an instant-read thermometer. Add more coals and remaining wood chips as needed during grilling.

Remove roast from grill. Cover with foil; let stand for 15 minutes. The temperature of the meat will rise 5 degree F during standing. To serve, slice pork.

Nutritional Readout: Calories 190, FAT 9 g, PROTEIN 24 g., CARB. 5.3 g. FIBER .01

Grilled Pesto Lamb Chops

Bright Mediterranean flavors bring hints of the middle East to these luscious chops.

Makes 4 servings

1 cup fresh basil leaves
1 tablespoon grated parmigiano
2 teaspoons pine nuts
2 cloves garlic, smashed
2 tablespoons Greek yogurt
4 4-ounce lamb chops
Kosher salt and freshly milled black pepper
1 tablespoon extra virgin olive oil

Position knife blade in food processor bowl; add basil, Parmigiano, pine nuts and garlic. Process until smooth. Transfer mixture to a small bowl; stir in yogurt. Cover and chill 30 minutes.

Heat grill, then coat grill rack with vegetable cooking spray Season chops with salt and pepper then cook 5minutes per side or until medium rare. Serve with a dollop of pesto on each chop. Garnish with fresh basil sprigs.

Nutritional information: 214 calories, FAT 9.8 g., PROTEIN 27.8 g., CARB 2.1 g., FIBER 1.2 g.

Super Easy Baked Ham

Start with a fully cooked ham, coat it with mustard and you'll have a treat that's delicious hot or cold.

Makes 12 servings

1 6 to 8 lb cooked ham, bone-in shank half
Ballpark yellow mustard to coat the outside.

Preheat oven to 350°F. and make sure the racks are all the way on the bottom so there is plenty of room for the ham.

Take ham out of wrapper and rinse it with cool water. Place ham in pan with large cut side down.. Make cross hatch mark in the skin and place it skin side up in a roasting pan. Coat with mustard.

Cook until internal temperature reaches 140 degrees. Set it aside to rest before carving.

Nutritional readout: 535 calories, FAT 39.7 g., PROTEIN 41.3g. CARB 4.3 g., FIBER 2.0 g

Branzino with Walnut Puree

Recipe courtesy California Walnut Board, Chef Ethan Stowell of Union in Seattle. A quick and satisfying supper. Before you get to The Marathon, skip the greens and just enjoy the fish. Makes 4 servings.

1 cup California walnut pieces, toasted a moment in a dry skillet
1/4 cup extra virgin olive oil, plus 2-3 tablespoons
2 tablespoons finely chopped fresh chives
2 whole branzino (or white sea bass) cut into fillets, 4 total
Kosher salt
Freshly ground black pepper

To make the walnut puree, combine the walnuts and 1/4 cup of olive oil in a food processor and process for about 1 minute, or until smooth (add more olive oil if needed). Scrape the walnut puree into a bowl and stir in the chives, and season with salt and pepper to taste. Set aside.

Rub the fish with 2-3 tablespoons of olive oil, and season both sides with salt and pepper. Just before you cook the fish, place about 2 tablespoons of the walnut puree in the center of 4 dinner plates. Grill the fish 2-3 minutes on each side. Place a fish fillet on each plate, over the walnut puree.

Nutritional readout: 482 calories, FAT 36.5 g., PROTEIN 35.8 g., CARB 4.0g. FIBER .6g

Seared Scallops with Gremolata

Choose large, meaty sea scallops for ease of preparation, and remember this gremolata, which is simply a Mediterranean mix of fresh herbs works well with other protein choices as well: lamb, chicken, turkey. Make the recipe work for you.

Makes 4 servings

1 1/2 lb. large sea scallops
sea salt and freshly milled black pepper to taste
1 tablespoon extra virgin olive oil, divided
1 shallot, minced
½ cup dry white wine
Juice and grated zest of 1 lemon
1 tablespoon minced Italian parsley
1 tablespoon minced chives
1 tablespoon minced basil

Season scallops with salt and pepper on a paper towel. Heat half the oil in a large skillet then sear the scallops until brown on the edges, about 3-4 minutes. Move t a warm dish.

Add remaining oil, shallots and sauté 1 minute, and then add wine, lemon, parsley, chives and basil. Heat 1 minute then pour over scallops and serve.

Nutritional readout: 175 calories, FAT 3.7 g., PROTEIN 28.8 g., CARB 4.3 g., FIBER .3 g.

Seared Cod with Browned Butter and Almonds

Any cold water firm fleshed fish will work with this recipe. You'll be getting lots of omega 3's and 6's as well as fantastic flavor.

Makes 4 servings

4 6-ounce cod fillets
Kosher salt and freshly milled black pepper to taste
3 tablespoons butter
¼ cup sliced almonds
Juice and grated zest of ½ lemon

Season fish with salt and pepper. Heat a skillet to medium high, and then add butter. Melt it then sauté the fish, until golden on each side, adding almonds the last minute. Add lemon, stir, and then plate the fish and pour the sauce.

Nutritional readout: 226 calories, FAT 9.8 g., PROTEIN 31.7 g., CARB 1.9 g., FIBER .8g.

Lemon Yellow Tail with Tomato-Dill Sauce

This popular Gulf of Mexico fish is a cousin to Amberjack, and mild flavored and wonderful with sauces. As always, substitute whatever you find in the case that's really fresh.

Makes 4 servings

4 6 ounce yellow tail fillets
2 tablespoons yellow mustard
Kosher salt and freshly milled black pepper to taste
2 tablespoons extra virgin olive oil
¼ cup minced green onions
1 plum tomato, minced
Juice and grated zest of 1 lemon
½ cup dry white wine
2 tablespoons butter

Rub mustard, salt and pepper over fish on both sides. Heat oil in a large skillet and sauté fish until golden, about 5 minutes. Remove to a warm plate. Add green onions, tomato and lemon to the pan and cook about 1 minute. Add wine and cook down by half. Swirl in butter to make a sauce, and pour over fish and serve.

Nutritional readout: 235 calories, FAT 8.2 g., PROTEIN 34.6 g., CARB 4.2 g., FIBER 0.6 g.

Curry Orange Salmon

Citrus and curry make a splendid sweet, sour hot and sassy flavor note for the ubiquitous salmon. Remember to buy only wild caught salmon, never farm raised.

Makes 4 servings

¼ cup chopped cilantro
3 tablespoons extra virgin olive oil, divided
1 tablespoon curry powder
Juice and grated zest of 1 orange
Salt and freshly milled black pepper to taste
1-1/2 pounds salmon sides
Lime wedges

Stir together cilantro, 1 tablespoon oil, curry, lime and salt and pepper. Paste it onto the fish. Heat remaining oil in a large skillet and sauté fish until golden, about 4 minutes. Serve with lime wedges.

Nutritional readout: 308 calories, FAT 16.6 g., PROTEIN 36.3 g., CARB 1.7 g., .3 g. FIBER

Grilled Salmon Provencal with Yogurt Sauce

Salmon steaks are great for this satisfying 10 minute dinner.

Makes 4 servings

½ cup Greek yogurt
2 garlic cloves, minced
Kosher salt and freshly milled black pepper to taste
4 6-ounce salmon steaks
2 tablespoons extra virgin olive oil
2 cups berry tomatoes, halved
3 tablespoons basil, cut chiffonade

Stir together yogurt, garlic and salt and pepper. Set it aside. Season tuna with salt and pepper. Heat a large skillet with oil and sauté tuna steaks until golden, about 3 minutes per side. Remove to a warm plate. Add tomatoes and basil to the pan and heat for 3 minutes or so until soft. Mound tuna and tomatoes on a plate and top with a dollop of yogurt.

Nutritional Readout: 256 calories, FAT 6.5 g., PROTEIN 43.1 g., CARB 4.8 g., FIBER 1.1 g

Bone Broth will strengthen your immune system.

Dr. Weston A. Price, the dentist who roamed the earth studying native cultures in the early part of the twentieth century was the first one to record the ravages of the Western diet in his book, Nutrition and Physical Degeneration, first published in 1939 and in continual publication since.

Dr. Price recorded cultures from the Amazon to the Arctic, noting the diets of native peoples before and after they'd been introduced to the so-called Western diet. He concluded that much of the so-called modern diet was impacting the health of people around the world.

"Life in all its fullness is mother nature obeyed," said Dr. Price. For a great resource and for sound nutritional advice log onto (www.westonaprice.org). See the website for dates for the annual conference which provides a wealth of information.

This basic broth recipe is found in traditional cultures from Eastern Europe to South America. We use this broth as the basis for soups, to start meals, and to build up our immune systems. Not only is it good for us, it also tastes good.

Bone Broth

I often buy chicken backs and beef neck bones and combine the two to make this healthy broth.

Makes about one gallon
2-4 pounds raw chicken or beef bones
2 tablespoons apple-cider vinegar
1 gallon water
1 onion, cut in chunks
1 head of garlic, broken into cloves and smashed

Simmer bones in water and vinegar at least 5 hours. The bones will soften, and the vinegar helps release minerals into the broth. When broth is cool, skim off fat, strain and store broth in zip locks in the freezer.

Nutritional Readout per cup: 55 calories, FAT 1.2 g., PROTEIN 5.1g. CARBS 0.5 g., FIBER 0.

Lemon Water

In the 1940's a craze swept outward from Hollywood and it was called "the Master Cleanse". Basically it was a fast that ordered people to drink lemon water with a shot of cayenne for days on end to detoxify their bodies.

Although, we do not recommend restricting yourself to lemon water alone, we do believe it is a healthy addition to the Silver Cloud Diet Detox.

1 8 ounce glass ice water
Juice of half a lemon
Whiff of cayenne
Stevia to sweeten

Stir and enjoy. You could drink four of these a day and you would not only lose weight but also build your immune system with the super charge of vitamin C you're getting.

Nutritional Readout: 1.3 calories, FAT 0, PROTEIN 0, CARBS .4 g, FIBER 0

Full Fat Chocolate Ice Cream

One of my particular weaknesses is ice cream. I might be able to eschew cakes and pies, even my beloved chocolate chip cookies, but ice cream? I don't think so.

I dug out my first cookbook and made a version of my favorite traditional custard ice cream, simply substituting Stevia for the sugar, and adding some fine European cocoa I'd brought home from my last trip.

I used the traditional method, and when it was made, the flavor was fantastic. You can substitute other flavorings for the cocoa: lemon zest and juice, orange, crushed coffee beans, a vanilla bean, smashed berries of your choice.

No doubt, the original REAL ice cream. All we've done is replace sugar with all natural stevia. You will thank me for this. Readers often tell me they buy a cookbook for one recipe. This is that recipe.

Makes 1 quart

15 minutes to cook custard
4 hours + to cure in the refrigerator
20 minutes to freeze in electric ice cream maker

4 large organic egg yolks
4 cups heavy cream
¼ cup best quality unsweetened cocoa
Pinch salt
8 -10 drop liquid stevia (or to taste)

Whip egg yolks and half the cream in a glass measure or bowl. Pour remaining cream, cocoa and salt in a heavy bottom saucepan and heat until cocoa is completely dissolved.

Pour custard and cocoa mixture together and whisk thoroughly. Cook until the custard coats the back of a spoon. Cover and refrigerate at least 4 hours. Pour the mixture into the ice cream canister and freeze in your ice cream maker.

Nutritional readout: 454 calories, FAT 47.3 g., PROTEIN 4.3 g., CARBS 6.2 g., FIBER, 8

Classic Custard

Here's a fool-proof dessert for you to make and refrigerate until you really need a sweet finish to dinner. It even works well as a snack. You can gild it further by a dollop of whipped cream if you wish.

Makes 6 servings

4 cups (1 quart) heavy cream
6 large eggs, separated
1/4 teaspoon cream tartar
1/4 teaspoon salt
6 packets sugar substitute (or to taste)
2 teaspoons vanilla extract
1 teaspoon almond extract
Ground cinnamon on top
Blueberries, strawberries, or raspberries for garnish

Preheat the oven to 325° F. Spritz a 4-quart casserole or 6 individual ramekins with buttery cooking spray and set it aside. Place a large pan with 1 inch of water in the middle of the lower rack of the oven to preheat.

Pour cream into a microwave safe bowl and heat at 100% power 4 minutes. Alternately, heat stovetop to just under the boil.

Meanwhile, beat egg whites with cream tartar and salt until soft peaks form.

In a large separate bowl, beat egg yolks with sweetener until well-blended then pour in hot cream and beat a moment. Season with vanilla and almond extracts. Fold beaten egg whites into this mixture.

Pour into prepared casserole or ramekins, top with a sprinkling of ground cinnamon, cover with buttered parchment

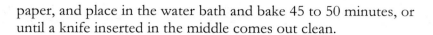

paper, and place in the water bath and bake 45 to 50 minutes, or until a knife inserted in the middle comes out clean.

Serve custard warm or cold in a dessert dish with a side of fresh berries. Top with whipped cream if you wish.

Nutritional readout: 289 calories, FAT 22 g., PROTEIN 10.2 g., CARB 10.9 g., FIBER .4 g

Cinnamon Soufflé

A perfect punctuation point to a divine dinner.Master soufflés and omelets and you're on the way to becoming a fabulous cook. This simple lovely soufflé makes a satisfying end to a rich country meal.

Choose the best cinnamon you can lay hands on for optimum flavor. For the best flavor, use your microplane and grate the cinnamon yourself from whole cinnamon sticks.

Makes 8 ½ cup servings

12 ounces cream cheese
16 ounces sour cream or crème fraiche
8 drops stevia (or up to 6 packets – to taste)
Pinch salt
½ teaspoon freshly grated cinnamon
8 large eggs, separated.

Separate the eggs. Heat oven to 300° F. Thoroughly mix cream cheese, sour cream, stevia, salt, cinnamon and egg yolks in a large bowl.

Beat egg whites. In the stand mixer, beat egg whites until stiff, then fold in the egg yolk mixture. Divide among ramekins, or in a large soufflé pan. Place ramekins on a baking sheet then bake until golden, brown and puffed (about 18 minutes for individuals and 45 minutes for the large one).

Serve immediately. Once you're in the marathon phase, add a side of raspberries

Nutritional readout: 333 calories, FAT 28.5g. PROTEIN 10.4g., CARBS 5.8g., FIBER 0.1g.

French Chocolate Cake (Flourless)

Serve warm or cold with whipped cream. The cream may be sweetened with stevia and dusted with cocoa powder before serving. For the Marathon phase, add a few berries on the side.

Makes 12 servings

½ cup Dutch Process European pure unsweetened cocoa
6 oz 70% cacao dark chocolate
1 cup unsalted butter
10 packets (or to taste) stevia
4 large eggs, separated

Preheat oven to 350° F. Line one 9-inch removable bottom cake tin with parchment paper and generously coat the paper with butter
Break the chocolate into pieces and melt it with butter and cocoa over hot water stirring with a rubber spatula.

Beat the egg yolks with the sugar substitute until light. Fold in the melted butter and chocolate mixture.

Beat egg whites until stiff peaks form. Fold into chocolate mixture. Pour into the prepared pan.

Bake at 350° degrees until a wooden pick inserted in center comes out clean, approximately 40 minutes.

Use a knife to separate the cake from the non-stick paper. Please observe that the cake is quite sticky!

Nutritional readout: 263 calories, FAT 23.2 g., PROTEIN 3.9 g., CARBS 9.8 g., FIBER 2.2 g.

Part III: The Silver Cloud Marathon: the road to good health, normal weight, and long and vigorous life

Join the marathon and you can expect to lose two to five pounds a week, you won't feel hungry, and you shouldn't suffer cravings. If you do, I'll tell you what to do about them too.

As I've said before, the human body is amazingly adaptable, and just as it adapted to an eating pattern that packed on the pounds and threatened your health, given a chance, your body can heal itself. All you have to do is cooperate a bit.

The marathon will reintroduce complex carbohydrates in a step wise fashion. After your week or two in detox, your body is now ready for the long haul. Whether you need to lose 20 pounds or 200, this marathon will get you there.

I promised you wouldn't have to count calories, or worry about fat every again, but you need to be aware of carbohydrates and reintroduce complex carbohydrates in an orderly way so that you don't undo the good work you've done in the Detox period.

Keep in mind that complex carbohydrates are whole vegetables, fruits and grains. Simple carbohydrates, such as sugars, flours, and processed foods are not on your food list. And actually should never be except for very special occasions.

OK. You can have a piece of cake on your birthday.

But the really remarkable thing about the Silver Cloud Diet plan is that once you've reset your body clock, given your body a rest from all the junk food you once craved, you will be amazed to discover that you may not even want that piece of cake.

Alright, I'm lying. You will want chocolate cake as long as you live, but at least you should restrict yourself to one tiny piece, even if it is your birthday.

Be patient with yourself. This change takes time. Some people are more addicted than others to chips, cookies, soda, and all the zillion and one bad-for-you foods. But the more you nourish your body with whole, organic foods, the less your body will be screaming for the bad stuff.

This time, you can really do it.

Diet   **Exercise**   **Attitude**

Remember, this is a tri-part system. The more you experience success on the Silver Cloud, the more success you will have. You've already succeeded at the Detox portion, I hope you've ramped up your exercise to the point that you are walking every day, and I'm sure your attitude is improving because you are making positive changes in your body. Aim for 10,000 steps a day. Buy a pedometer. This isn't as hard as it sounds.

What's next? You will have plenty of energy, you will feel good, you will look good and you will achieve your dietary goals.

Add a simple weight lifting regimen to your week. 2-3 times a week, lift 5 pound weights, in a program to increase your upper body strength. Go to a gym, hire a personal trainer, or buy an appropriate video to guide you. If you're a beginner, start here: http://www.ehow.com/how_5199034_start-weight-training-women.html

The Silver Cloud Diet Marathon is a progression into a broad and varied diet of organic whole and unprocessed foods for health, weight loss, and long life.

Five Easy Steps to Dieting Success with The Silver Cloud

- Pay attention to everything you eat.
- Learn to control the portions
- Drink plenty of water. At least 64 ounces, including tea and coffee
- Add a squeeze of lemon juice and shot of cayenne for the full detox effect
- Eat 5 meals a day.
- 2 eggs for breakfast
- 4-5 ounces of fish or meat twice a day
- Small snacks morning and evening, nutrient dense cheese, nuts, olives, jerky, ham,or turkey
- Be mindful of what your body is telling you.
- Try to get 8 hours sleep every night
- Exercise by vigorous walking at least 15 minutes every day. Add exercise time and rigor as you are able. Work up to 10,000 steps if you can. (Buy a pedometer. We like the Omron.)
- Take proactive steps to reduce stress in your life: yoga, meditation, removal of stressful people in your life

At first, you may notice that paying attention to everything you eat seems like a chore, but soon it will become second nature. Make a point of sitting down to eat, away from your desk, away from the telephone, away from the television. Be mindful of the food you put in your mouth.

This diet is made up of the finest, purest foods there are. It is a luxury to eat this way. You deserve the very best. This diet makes that happen. Make a conscious choice not to eat junk food. Eliminate white flour and sugar from your diet in all combinations.

Portion control is perhaps the biggest challenge for those of us who have been living on the so-called Western diet in which the super-sized portions have created a nation of overfed, undernourished people. If you learn to manage your portions, you won't have to count calories. Buy yourself a scale and weigh meats and cheeses to get accustomed to serving sizes. This will help you when you go out to eat where most so-called portion are at least twice and sometimes three times the amount of food needed for nourishment.

***3 ounces of meat is about the size of a deck of cards
1 ounce of cheese is about the size of a domino***

Start your day with a hot cup of tea or coffee. This stimulates the digestive system and will help you to feel full faster. If you have trouble drinking the amount of water you need, buy yourself a 64 ounce sports bottle and fill it up. By the end of the day, make sure you have drunk every drop.

Drinking water before a meal also helps you to feel fuller. Try this in a restaurant. Ask for water when you sit down, and drink down the whole glass before the food arrives.

Making your metabolism work better and regulating your glucose depends on regular small servings of high protein, high fat meals. This will stop your cravings in their tracks. You won't get those desperate urges for junk food from the machine or the deli down on the corner.

Becoming mindful of your body is often a new thing for people who have had years of overweight. Many people stop looking at themselves in the mirror. They don't ever experience their body as being "empty".

They confuse hypoglycemia – which is a status wherein your blood sugars have dropped precipitously, warning you that you're about to go into shock – with hunger. A body that is well nourished and receiving sufficient protein on a regular basis throughout the day will regulate itself.

You will burn fat. You will never feel hungry. You can trust your body which, given a chance, can regulate itself. You will soon cast long, loving looks at yourself in the mirror, because you will look GREAT.

Exercise: It's Easier Than You Think

Now that many of us are planted in front of a computer for 8 or more hours a day, the notion of exercise may seem impossible. But, if you stop and think of your normal day's activities you may see how you can tuck in some exercise with out too much effort.

If you sit at a computer terminal, get up and walk for 5 minutes every hour. Try running up and down a flight of stairs – just for the fun of it.

Walk it Off.

You don't have to go crazy here, just take a brisk 15 minute walk sometime during the day. Walk your dogs. Walk on your lunch hour. Take the stairs instead of the elevator. Park in the spot FARTHEST from the Mall. If you have an exercise bike in the basement, jump on it for 15 minutes. Whatever you do, try to get your heart rate up and pounding. Try to walk 10,000 steps during your day.

Strength Training.

You may be getting strength training in your daily life. Got a toddler you're carrying around? Hauling groceries in the house on a daily basis? Pushing a heavy vacuum cleaner? Gardening? All these exercises build strength. But for a more focused exercise plan, give yourself 15 minutes a day – OK, go ahead. Multitask. Watch the news on TV while you're making yourself stronger. Use a couple 3 pound weights and do some lifts and pull ups. Use an exercise rope and do some bicep curls, or front raises. Start out doing 10 and work up to 25 reps.

Lay on the floor and do some old fashioned sit ups. 10 to start and up to 20. Just feel the burn and keep at it. You'll make yourself stronger.

The quickest way to get started is to hire a personal trainer for a few sessions. Work with your trainer to establish a routine that works for you.

Sleep it off

Get a full 8 hours of rest. Every night. No matter what. Feeling insomniac? Try drinking 2 tablespoons cream.

What you need to do and why

Assess yourself. Have you lost 5 to 15 pounds? Has your waist size dropped 2-4 inches? Checked your BMI? Make sure it's on the downward run. http://www.cdc.gov/healthyweight/assessing/bmi/adult_bmi/english.

Is your waist measurement over 35 inches – for women, 40 inches for men? If so, you are still in the obese category and should stick with the Full Fat Fast, the Silver Cloud Detox Plan another week or so or until you're out of the danger zone.

We've had patients who stayed on the Detox phase for months. No harm done. Eating out for lunch after a 2 egg breakfast is easy. Order a chop, a steak, a fish steak or fillet. Some shrimp. See? Not so hard.

Case study:

When Paul came to see me six weeks ago, he was 120 pounds overweight. His cardiologist told him he was headed for myocardial infarction, aka a heart attack. He began the Detox program, and ultimately stayed on it for a little over one month. In 35 days, Paul lost 40 pounds and happily moved to the marathon phase to continue his weight loss program.
When you've graduated from detox. Here's how to start your own marathon, to keep yourself on that Silver Cloud.

FOODS TO ADORE

Fats	extra virgin olive oil, butter, unrefined flax oil, coconut oil, fresh lard, foie gras, nuts (walnuts, pecans, brazil nuts, and hazelnuts)
Proteins	organic or grass fed beef, pork, veal, lamb, game, chicken, turkey, duck and other fowl (where possible). Chicken or veal liver, nitrate free bacon and sausage, all seafood from cold, deep water (including codfish, halibut, and salmon), shellfish, and eggs
Dairy	butter, raw milk cheeses, organic full fat light or whipping cream, Greek yogurt, buttermilk, heavy and sour cream from pasture-fed cows.
vegetables	Salad vegetables: 2-3 cups arugula, cabbage,

and fruits	celery, chicory, chives, cucumber daikon, endive, escarole, fennel, jicama, lettuces, mache, mushrooms, parsley, peppers, radicchio, radishes, scallions, sorrel, spinach, sprouts of all kinds, tomato, watercress Cooked vegetables: 1 cup added to 2 cups of salad per day Artichokes, whole or hearts, asparagus, bamboo shoots, bean sprouts, beet greens, bok choy, broccoli, broccoli rabe, Brussels sprouts, cabbage, cauliflower, celery root, chard, collard greens, dandelion greens, eggplant, hearts of palm, kale, kohlrabi, leeks, okra, onion, pumpkin, rhubarb, sauerkraut, snow peas, spaghetti squash, string or wax beans, summer squash, tomato, turnip, water chestnuts, zucchini Berries, ½ cup then later add ½ stone fruits (pears, peaches, plums, nectarines)
Beverages	water, lemon water, coffee, tea (at least 64 ounces a day) bottled waters of all kinds without added sugars. Herb tea, broth, club soda and seltzers without added sugars. Use stevia or Splenda to sweeten. Low carb cocktails
Condiments	Kosher or sea salt, black and red pepper, best quality balsamic vinegar, apple cider vinegar, rice wine vinegar, mayonnaise, mustards, soy sauce, fish sauce. crumbled bacon, grated hard cheeses,

	minced hard cooked egg, sautéed mushrooms, spices and herbs, prepared salad dressings with no carbs. Caponata, horseradish, pesto, pickles without sugar, tamari, Tabasco, tapenade, Worcestershire sauce, shiritake or Miracle Noodles

Be a label reader. Many so-called "diet foods" are loaded with carbohydrates. Don't be fooled. Read the fine print. If a food product has more than 10 grams carb, put it back.

FOODS TO ABHOR

Fats	highly processed vegetable oils like canola or soybean, margarine, vegetable shortening. All trans-fats often found in processed foods and snacks.
Proteins	processed meats
Dairy	processed cheeses, reduced or non-fat dairy products
Carbohydrates	any highly processed carbohydrate, white flour or anything made from white flour (including bread, cookies, crackers, pastas, and dry cereals), high fructose corn syrups, refined sugars, irradiated or genetically modified grains, chocolate mixed with sugar in any form
Beverages	soda, full strength fruit juices, bear, wine, rice milk

Condiments	catsup, commercial baking powder, MSG, artificial flavors, additives and colors

Remember to select foods that are sustainable, organic if possible and whole and unprocessed all the time.

Part I of the Marathon.

Keep carbs to net 20 grams per day.
Start with 3 cups of salad greens, or two cups salad + 1 cup cooked vegetables (from approved list) for the first week.

Enjoy full fat, raw milk aged cheese – up to 4 ounces a day, a handful of olives and a half an avocado every day. Dress your salads with extra virgin olive oil and vinegar or lemon juice.

And remember you don't need to measure meats, fish, or fowl. Just eat as much as you wish, including that yummy skin and fat. Try to become really aware of when you are full. Be mindful. Pay attention. Eat only until you are satisfied, not until you are stuffed.

After a week or so, add back more vegetables and fruits. By now you should be eating 9 servings of vegetables and fruits a day. So long as your weight continues to drop you can stay at this level.

Once you've come with 10 pound of your goal weight, add back a few complex carbohydrates. Say a cup of oatmeal for breakfast, or a piece of multigrain bread for lunch.

Always monitor your weight and should you hit a plateau that holds for several weeks, simply give yourself a week of the Detox level again, and you'll be back on track.

If you wish, check the nutrient data from the U.S. government. http://www.nal.usda.gov/fnic/foodcomp/search/

Ask.com has a good, free online carb counter. Or, buy yourself a carb counter book. We recommend Dr. Atkins' New Carbohydrate Gram Counter (Paperback) only 4.95 from Amazon.

Try squeezing lemon into ice water with a bit of artificial sweetener and a whiff of cayenne for your own kicked up beverage. Avoid diet sodas. Some studies have shown that they "trick" the body to behaving as if real sugar had been consumed. Don't risk it.

Include these flavorful nutrient dense additives for snacks as needed: 10 olives, half a Haas avocado. 2-3 tablespoons lemon or lime juice, pork skins, string cheese, beef jerky.

Once your marathon is well under way, you may add more salad, other vegetables, fresh cheeses, seeds and nuts. Berries, legumes, fruits other than berries, some starchy vegetables and whole grains.

Be mindful of your weight and if you hit a plateau, back up to the stage of the marathon or detox phase where you succeeded before by cutting out any of the foods listed above and your weight loss should begin again.

And remember to keep moving. Try to get in 10,000 steps a day. Keep a positive attitude and you will succeed.

This time you can really do it.

Buy your produce from a farmer's market for best flavor and nutrition.

For breakfast, check out all the egg recipes if you like variety. Add breakfast meats as you wish, nitrate free bacon and sausages are fine.

This grid tells you *categories* you should aim for. Recipes follow. And remember to drink 64 ounces of fluids without *any* sugar daily and to do at least 15 minutes of walking to jumpstart your marathon.

Tea and coffee are fine. Sweeten with stevia and add cream if you wish.

Read labels ardently. If any prepared food product has more than 10 carb grams, just put it back, no matter how the product is billed. You may subtract fiber from the carbs but the NET result should always be 10 carb grams OR LESS.

Want to know what a serving is?

½ apple
8 spears asparagus
½ Haas avocado
1/2 cup berries: black, blue, raspberries and strawberries
2/3 cup cooked broccoli
¼ cup cantaloupe or honeydew
1 cup cauliflower
1/3 cup cooked corn, on or off the cob
1 kiwi
1/3 cup cooked legumes: kidney beans, chickpeas, lentils and limas
½ cup cooked oatmeal
1/3 cup cooked onions
½ cup cooked red peppers
¼ cup cooked brown rice
1 cup cooked pumpkin
¾ cup cooked spinach

2/3 cup summer squash
1 tangerine
1 medium tomato

Think of it this way. In the first phase of the marathon, you will begin by aiming for 20 carbohydrate grams limit per day for the first period. You will lose 2-5 pounds per week.

Once you've come within 15 pounds of goal weight, you can ramp it up to 40 carbohydrate grams per day, and you can expect to lose 1 to 2 pounds per week.

Once you are within 5 pounds of goal weight. Push it up to 60 carbohydrate grams and include whole wheat bread (1 slice) brown rice (1/2 cup) or whole wheat pasta (1/2 cup). Now is when you can enjoy that occasional piece of cake or chocolate chip cookie. You will probably not lose much weight at 60 grams carbohydrate but now you know what you should be doing for the rest of your life.

Your appetite will change. You will look at a plate of food with a different eye. You won't even consider that pile of pasta. You'll just enjoy a half cup. Buckets of rice? I don't' think so. ½ cup once you're near your goal weight. This will not be hard. I promise. You are on your Silver Cloud for life.

The great thing about the marathon is that you have changed your habits; you now get it about what it takes to live a long and healthy life. Design your own life and your own eating plan.

Just choose whole unprocessed foods, organic if possible. Buy your meat and fish from vendors who will tell you where the meat came from and if the fish is "wild caught". Shop farmer's markets and local vendors. Eat as close the ground as you can.

This time you can really do it

The Counter Intuitive Food List

Shorthand to Portion Sizes to stay on your Silver Cloud.

Shop for whole, unprocessed foods at all times. Organic if possible.

Stay away from processed foods and most "diet" foods which are often loaded with chemicals and unhealthy filler.

Meat and Beans: Aim for at least 3-4 servings each day. Choose fresh, unprocessed meats and nitrate free bacon and sausages whenever possible. No restriction on portions except for beans.

Item	One serving equals	That's about the size of
Meat & Tofu	2-3 oz cooked beef, poultry, fish, tofu	Billiard ball
Beans	1/2 cup cooked beans, split peas, legumes	Billiard ball
Nuts & Seeds	Hand Full	One Hand Full

Fruits and Vegetables: Aim 5-9 total servings each day. Choose fresh fruits and veggies whenever possible.

Examples	One serving equals	That's about the size of
Raw fruit	1/2 cup raw, canned, frozen berries and fruit	Billiard ball
Dried fruit	1/4 cup raisins, prunes, apricots	An egg

Raw vegetables	1 cup leafy greens, cukes, and others	Baseball
Cooked vegetables	1/2 cup cooked broccoli, asparagus etc.	Billiard ball

Dairy: Aim for 2-3 servings of calcium-rich foods each day. Choose light or heavy cream, sour cream. Avoid low fat or fat free milk. Pick full-fat raw milk cheeses. Avoid cheese food and all low fat or non fat cheeses. Look for raw milk full fat cheeses.

Examples	One serving equals	That's about the size of
Cheese	1 ounce full fat or 1 thin slice of cheese	A pair of dice
Milk	½ cup cream	Baseball

Fats & Oils: Eat natural fats and cold-pressed oils as needed. Choose heart-healthy fats whenever possible. No solid margarine or vegetable oils which are known as trans-fats. Expeller nut oils, extra virgin olive oil, coconut oil, and sesame oil are all great.

Examples	One serving equals	That's about the size of
Fat & Oil	1 -2 tablespoons unprocessed oil or butter	Spread through the day

Bread	1 ounce (1 small slice, 1/2 bagel, 1/2 bun, whole wheat and mixed grains)	Index card
Cooked Grains	1/2 cup cooked oats, brown rice, pasta	Index card

Whole Grains: Once you've reached the last leg of the marathon, where you are running full out, and are within 10 pounds of your goal weight, add back this category. Aim for 2-3 servings each day.   The recipes listed below are simply great ideas for you to build on. Remember to eat all the protein and fat you want, but STOP eating when you're full. Don't gorge yourself.

Add back those complex carbohydrates as your weight normalizes. 9 servings of complex carbohydrates a day
(that's about 4-1/2 cups).

Start off with leafy green veggies and berries, then gradually add in fruits and finally whole grains. You can find great recipes in magazines and books, just read the nutritional readout and watch out for hidden carbs. They are your enemy now and forever more.

In the beginning, restrict yourself to fewer than 20 carbohydrate grams a DAY.

Thai Beef Lettuce Wraps

The brightly flavored recipes of Thailand have been widely adored in this country. No wonder. Yum.

1 pound ground sirloin
1 tablespoon dark sesame oil, divided
2 tablespoons minced fresh ginger
¼ cup soy sauce
1 tablespoon rice vinegar
½ teaspoon dark sesame oil
½ teaspoon red pepper flakes
½ cup minced green onions
¼ cup chopped fresh cilantro
3 tablespoons chopped fresh mint
8 iceberg lettuce leaves
1 Kirby cucumber, cut into fine slices

Heat a large skillet, film it with sesame oil, and then add beef and ginger. Sauté until beef is cooked through, about 5 minutes. Stir in soy sauce, rice vinegar, remaining sesame oil, and red pepper. Cook about a minute. Off heat add onions, cilantro and mint. Divide among lettuce leaves and serve, with sliced cucumbers.

Nutritional readout: 158 calories, FAT 5.5 g., PROTEIN 23.7 g., CARB 5 g., FIBER 1.3 g.

Butter Lettuce Wraps with Peanut Sauced Shrimp and Mango

Wrap lettuce around most anything you used to use as a sandwich filling and it will taste good and be good for you.

Makes 16 servings

1/3 cup flaked unsweetened coconut
1-1/2 pounds chopped cooked shrimp
2 cups diced mango
Juice and grated zest from 3 limes
2 tablespoons finely chopped fresh mint
16 butter lettuce leaves
½ cup bottled peanut sauce
2 tablespoons chopped roasted almonds

Cook coconut in a small skillet just until fragrant, and then add to a bowl holding shrimp, mango, lime juice and zest, and mint. Toss and divide among lettuce leaves.

Stir remaining lime juice into peanut sauce and drizzle over shrimp. Fold leaves into diaper-fold and serve.

Nutritional readout: 84 calories, FAT 3g. PROTEIN 7.1 g., CARB 7.1 g., FIBER .8 g.

Chipotle Scallop Lettuce Wraps

Almost anything for a sandwich tastes great in a lettuce wrap. This goes for those "wraps" for sale everywhere sold in diaper folded flour tortillas (ugh). The flavor of these yummy shrimps in crisp butter lettuce is superior on all fronts. Enjoy.

Makes 4 servings

1 tablespoon cumin seeds
1 teaspoon chili powder
Sea salt and freshly milled black pepper to taste
1-1/2 cups large scallops
2 tablespoons extra virgin olive oil
2 cloves garlic, smashed
½ cup minced red onion
4 large butter lettuce leaves
½ cup chopped cilantro
Juice and grated zest from 1 lime
4 teaspoons sour cream
4 tablespoons chipotle salsa

Combine cumin, chili powder, salt and pepper. Toss shrimp in this mixture. Heat oil in a large skillet. Add garlic and onion and cook a moment, then add shrimp and cook until opaque and golden, about 3 minutes. Divide among lettuce leaves then top each with cilantro, lime juice and zest, sour cream and salsa. Fold and enjoy.

Nutritional readout: 272 calories,   FAT11.2 g., PROTEIN 35.4 g., CARB 5.5 g., FIBER .09 g.

Pan Grilled Fish with Chermoula

Moroccans use this brightly flavored sauce with meat, fish, and shrimp. Take your pick. The results are the same. Fantastic!

Makes 4 servings

2 garlic cloves, smashed
½ teaspoon kosher salt
¼ cup extra virgin olive oil
Juice and grated zest of 1 lemon
2 tablespoons EACH: parsley and cilantro
1 teaspoon smoked paprika
½ teaspoon EACH: ground cumin, coriander, red pepper
1-1/2 pounds fish fillet or large peeled shrimp. (Even chicken or lamb)

Combine garlic and salt with a fork to make a paste, add oil, lemon, parsley, cilantro paprika, cumin, coriander and red pepper. Smear this paste on surfaces of the fish or meat. Cook on an olive oil coated pan or grill.

Nutritional readout: 282 calories, FAT 13.6 g., PROTEIN 23.9 g., CARB 4.4 g.,   FIBER .5 g.

Gingered Tilapia with Baby Spinach

On the table in 10 minutes and only 3 grams carbohydrate. Woo hoo.

Makes 4 servings

4 tilapia (or other mild fish) fillets, 6 oz. ea.
2 tablespoons freshly grated ginger root
Kosher salt and black pepper to taste
1-1/2 tablespoons extra virgin olive oil
1 small onion, minced
6 cups (2 packages) baby spinach
¼ cup chicken broth
¼ cup dry white wine

Rub fish fillets with ginger, salt and pepper. Heat oil in a large skillet over medium-high heat. Cook fish 2-3 minutes on each side, or until opaque. Remove from the pan and keep warm.

Film the pan with additional oil and cook onions and remaining ginger for 1 minute. Increase heat to high, and then add spinach, season with additional salt and pepper, chicken broth and wine. Cook 3 minutes or until wilted.

Serve fish on a bed of spinach and garnish with a lemon wedge.

Nutritional readout: 233 calories, FAT 8 g, PROTEIN 35 g, CARBOHYDRATE 3 g., FIBER 1 g.

Sole a la Bonne Femme

Got to hand it to the French. They eat well, and as well all understand, it's the reason French women always seem to be thin. Although the recipe calls for flounder fillet, substitute the freshest fish in your fish monger's case. Pick what you love.

Makes 4 servings in less than 20 minutes

4 flounder (or other) fish fillets, about 1 pound
Kosher salt and cracked black pepper
1 cup dry white wine
3 tablespoons butter
2 tablespoons shallots or green onions, minced + more for garnish
½ lb. sliced chanterelle (or button) mushrooms
¼ cup heavy cream
1 large egg yolk

Heat oven to 350°. Butter a baking dish generously then salt and pepper the fish and lay it in the dish. Pour wine over and bake covered about 10 minutes, or just until cooked through. Pour the pan juices into a saucepan with butter, shallots and mushrooms. Heat to boiling. Meanwhile whisk cream and egg yolk together then add to the sauce. To serve, pool sauce in a dinner sauce and add fish fillets. Garnish with minced shallots and serve.

Nutritional Readout: 349 calories, FAT 22 g., PROTEIN 23 g., CARB 3.3g. FIBER .02 g

Sautéed Shrimp on Red Cabbage with Parsley Sauce

Don't you just love One Dish Dinners?

Makes 4 servings

6 tablespoons extra virgin olive oil, divided
1 medium red cabbage, shredded (about 2 pounds)
1/2 cup dry red wine
6 tablespoons unsalted butter
1 tablespoon minced onion
1 garlic clove, minced
4 tablespoons flat-leaf parsley, finely chopped
1-1/2 pounds large peeled shrimp

Heat 2 tablespoons oil in a large skillet and add cabbage and a pinch of salt. Cook, until cabbage begins to melt, then add wine and cook and reduce 2-3 minutes more. Reduce heat to low, cover and cook until cabbage is tender, about 30 minutes. Adjust seasonings with salt. Transfer to a serving plate and cover.

Meanwhile, melt butter in a saucepan, add onion and garlic and cook until soft, about 3 minutes. Remove from the heat and stir in parsley. Season with salt and remaining oil and set it aside.

Heat 2 tablespoons oil in the skillet over medium heat. Cook shrimp just until it looks opaque, abut 3 minutes. Season with salt and freshly milled black pepper.

To serve, mound cabbage on a plate and arrange shrimp around it, drizzling with parsley sauce.

Nutritional readout: 304 calories, FAT 1.22 g, PROTEIN 19.6 g., CARB 9.6, FIBER 2.47 g

Grilled Chili Shrimp with Avocado Orange Salsa

On the table in under 15 minutes, this flavorful Southwestern lunch is easy to make and really delicious.

Makes 4 servings

1-1/2 pounds large, peeled shrimp

Mix together:

½ teaspoon ground cumin
1 teaspoon chili powder
 Kosher salt and fresh ground black pepper to taste

Avocado salsa:

1 large ripe Haas avocado, peeled, deseeded and chopped
½ cup minced cilantro
2 cloves garlic, smashed
2 tablespoons minced green onion
2 tablespoons minced tomato
 Juice and grated zest of one orange
2 tablespoons extra virgin olive oil

Dredge shrimp in cumin, chili powder, salt and pepper. Toss salsa ingredients together. Heat oil in a large skillet and sauté shrimp until opaque and golden, about 3 minutes. To serve, mound salsa on a plate and top with shrimp.

Nutritional readout: 242 calories, FAT 12.6 g., PROTEIN 28.2 g., CARB 5.4 g.,   FIBER 2.7 g.

Warm Salmon Salad with Caper Dressing

Quick as a wink and only 5 g. carb.

Makes 4 servings

1 head butter lettuce
1 1-lb. salmon fillet (about 1-1/4 inches thick)
1/2 teaspoon freshly ground black pepper
2 thick slices yellow onion
1/2 teaspoon dried or fresh dill weed
1 rib celery with leaves, minced

Caper Dressing:

2 tablespoons mayonnaise
2 tablespoons lemon juice + zest from 1/2 lemon
2 tablespoons water
1 tablespoon capers, drained

Line the bottom of the steamer rack with one lettuce leaf, then place the salmon, skin side down on the lettuce. Season with pepper. Arrange onions around the fish. Sprinkle with dill. Cover and steam over boiling water 10-18 minutes, or until the fish is cooked through and opaque*. Don't overcook the fish. Once it loses its translucent look in the center, remove it to a plate.

While the fish and vegetables are cooking, use a fork to whisk the dressing ingredients together.

Remove and discard the skin and bones from the cooked fish and break the fish into bite sized chunks. Add chopped celery. Toss with the dressing.

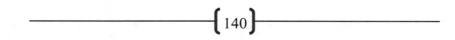

To serve, arrange lettuce leaves on dinner plates, and divide the salad equally among 4 servings. Garnish each serving with a twist of lemon.

*In a hurry, steam the fish on lettuce leaf in the microwave.
Done in 3-4 minutes. Easy peezy.

Nutritional readout: 303 calories, FAT 20.8 g, PROTEIN 24.1 g., CARB .5 g., FIBER 1.3 g

Artichokes, Capers, 0lives, Lemon Zest, and Salmon on Spaghetti Squash

In Italy a no-cook pasta sauce is known as salsa cruda, and makes a wonderful one-dish dinner. In this version, the combination of artichokes, olives, capers, and lemon zest is not only beautiful, but bold in flavor.

Makes 4 servings.

1 spaghetti squash

Salsa Cruda

1 (6-ounce) jar artichoke hearts, drained
1/4 cup drained and rinsed capers
1/2 cup pitted and chopped Kalamata olives
juice and zest of 1 lemon
1 16 ounce can salmon, drained
1/4 cup extra-virgin olive oil
freshly ground black pepper to taste
1/2 cup chopped fresh flat-leaf parsley leaves

Prick squash with a fork, then transfer to the microwave and cook for 10-12 minutes. Allow it to cool a few minutes then, cut in half. Remove seeds, then, using a fork, strip out spaghetti squash strings into a large serving bowl. Toss with salsa cruda ingredients. Garnish with chopped parsley leaves.

Nutritional readout: 403 calories, FAT 26.6 g., PROTEIN 22.1 g., CARB 14.9 g., FIBER 3.2 g

Dijon Egg and Salmon Salad

Here's one of those flavor hits that has everything: sweet, hot, bitter, salty, and crunchy in every bite. Served icy cold, it's a terrific lunch.

Makes 2 servings

2 large eggs, hard cooked, peeled, and finely chopped
1 cup canned salmon, drained
1/4 cup strawberries, chopped
2 tablespoons minced red onion
grated zest of 1 lemon (about 1 teaspoon)
1/4 cup toasted*, slivered almonds
3 tablespoons mayonnaise
2 tablespoons Dijon mustard
1/2 teaspoon freshly milled black pepper
6 leaves red tipped lettuce
1 cup radish sprouts
radishes for garnish

Stir together the chopped eggs, tuna, strawberries, onion, lemon zest, almonds, mayonnaise and mustard. Season to taste with freshly milled black pepper. Cover and refrigerate until serving time.

To serve, spread egg-tuna salad onto a piece of ruffled red lettuce and sprouts. Serve garnished with radishes. As many as you want.

Nutritional readout: 403 calories, FAT 27g. PROTEIN 33 g., CARB 10 g., FIBER 4 g.

Coq au Vin

The Classic French Dish made famous by Julia Child in the sixties is still fabulous for those on the Silver Cloud.

Makes 8 servings

1/2 lb bacon slices, coarsely chopped
20 pearl onions, peeled, or 1 large yellow onion, sliced
1 chicken, 4 lb, cut into serving pieces, or 3 lbs chicken parts, excess fat trimmed, skin ON
6 garlic cloves, peeled
Salt and pepper to taste
2 cups chicken stock
2 cups red wine (pinot noir, burgundy, or zinfandel)
2 bay leaves
Several fresh thyme sprigs
Several fresh parsley sprigs
1/2 lb button mushrooms, trimmed and roughly chopped
2 tablespoons butter
Chopped fresh parsley for garnish

Brown bacon on medium high heat in a Dutch oven big enough to hold the chicken, until golden. minutes. Remove the cooked bacon; add onions and chicken, skin side down. Brown the chicken well, on all sides. Halfway through the browning, add the garlic and sprinkle the chicken with salt and pepper.

Spoon off any excess fat. Add the chicken stock, wine, and herbs. Add back the bacon. Lower heat to a simmer. Cover and cook for 20 minutes, or until chicken is tender and cooked through. Remove chicken and onions to a separate platter. Remove the bay leaves, herb sprigs, garlic, and discard. Add mushrooms to the remaining liquid and turn the heat to high. Boil quickly and reduce the liquid by three fourths until it becomes thick and saucy. Lower the heat, stir in the butter. Return the chicken and onions to the pan to reheat and coat with sauce. Adjust seasoning. Garnish with parsley and serve.

` Nutritional readouts: 388 calories, FAT 5.9 g., PROTEIN 23.8 g., CARB 14.5 g., FIBER 2.10 g.

Chicken Breast in a Kalamata Caper Sauce

Boring chicken breasts need a lot of help. A shot of capers in a tomato pool is a good beginning. Plus it's on the table in less than 15 minutes. Yeah.

Makes 4 servings

4 boneless, skinless chicken breasts (4 oz each)
2 tablespoons Italian breadcrumbs
2 teaspoons extra virgin olive oil
¾ cup prepared salsa
½ diced plum tomato
½ cup diced zucchini
2 tablespoons seedless kalamata olives
2 teaspoons capers

Pound chicken breast between sheets of wax paper to a uniform ½-inch thickness. Sprinkle with breadcrumbs.

Heat oil in a large skillet and sauté chicken until golden, about 2 minutes on each side. Add a splash of water, cover and cook until done through, about 6 minutes.

Stir salsa, tomato, zuke, olives and capers together.

To serve arrange chicken on a plate and top with salsa.

Nutritional readout: 245 calories, FAT 5.1 g., PROTEIN 40.1 g., CARB 5.3 g., FIBER .6 g.

Easy Roast Chicken Thighs and Asparagus

Simple and satisfying, this one dish dinner goes together in a hurry. And check out the carb count, fewer than 8.

Makes 4 servings

2 garlic cloves
3 tablespoons extra virgin olive oil, divided
2 tablespoons fresh lemon juice, divided
8 chicken thighs with skin (about 1 3/4 pounds)
2 tablespoons unsalted butter, divided
1/2 cup chicken broth
1 teaspoon fresh or dried oregano
12 spears asparagus
Accompaniment: lemon wedges and parsley

Preheat oven to 450°. Mince garlic with a pinch of salt, then whisk together with 2 tablespoons oil, 1 tablespoon lemon juice, 1/2 teaspoon salt, and 1/4 teaspoon pepper. Pat chicken dry and coat with lemon-garlic mixture.

Heat 1 tablespoon butter and remaining tablespoon oil in a 12-inch heavy skillet over medium-high heat and brown chicken in 2 batches, skin side down, until golden and crisp, then remove to a baking dish, skin side up. Arrange asparagus alongside chicken.Pour off fat from skillet. Add broth and remaining tablespoon lemon juice and boil until reduced by half, about 2 minutes. Whisk in remaining tablespoon butter and oregano, and then pour over chicken and asparagus.

Roast chicken in oven until cooked through, about 20 minutes. Add a grating of freshly milled black pepper and serve, garnished with parsley and lemon wedges.

Nutritional Readout: 467 calories, FAT 33.3 g., PROTEIN 35.6 g., CARB 7.8 g., FIBER 1.3 g.

Chicken Thighs in a Mushroom Sauce

Meatier thighs have a great flavor and if you buy them boneless and skinless, they're oh so easy to deal with. On the table in under 15.

Makes 4 servings

2 cups chicken broth
¼ cup tomato paste
1 teaspoon dried rubbed sage
Kosher salt and freshly milled black pepper to taste
4 skinless, boneless chicken thighs
4 teaspoons Italian-seasoned breadcrumbs
1 tablespoon extra virgin olive oil
½ pound sliced baby bella mushrooms
4 green onions, thinly sliced on the diagonal

Combine broth with tomato paste, sage, salt and pepper, Set aside.

Sprinkle chicken with additional salt and pepper then breadcrumbs. Heat oil in a large skillet then cook 2-3 minutes per side. Add mushroom and brown them for 2 minutes, then add broth mixture. Cover and cook until chicken is done, about 10 minutes. Sprinkle with green onions and serve.

Nutritional readout: 260 calories, FAT 4.9 g., PROTEIN 44.1 g., CARB 9.2 g., FIBER 2.2 g.

Basil Parsley Chicken Salad

My hootsie-tootsie gourmet grocer sells organic roast chickens. I buy those fabulous birds and do many things with them. This vaguely French salad is one of my faves. Feel free to toss in other leafy greens of your choice, celery leaves, baby spinach, and mixed greens. This is a yummy lunch served over a bed of spring greens or wrapped in a butter lettuce leaf.

Makes 4 servings

1-1/2 cup cooked chicken, chopped
¼ cup basil, cut chiffonade
½ cup minced celery
¼ minced green onion
¼ cup chopped Italian parsley
2 tablespoons chopped sweet red peppers
½ cup mayonnaise
2 tablespoons Greek yogurt
Kosher salt and freshly milled black pepper to taste

Mix ingredients in a medium bowl, cover and refrigerate. Serve on a bed of spring greens. Or in a lettuce wrap.

Nutritional readout: 165 calories, FAT 7.2 g.,   PROTEIN 20 g., CARB 3.8 g., FIBER .7 g.

Feta-Stuffed Chicken

Feta is a full-flavored cheese that can be used in small amounts. Here it's mixed with a little cream cheese (lowering the carbohydrate content even more) and used as a stuffing for chicken.

Makes 4 servings

1/4 cup crumbled basil-and-tomato feta cheese (1 ounce)*

2   Tablespoons cream cheese (1 ounce)

4   skinless, boneless chicken breast halves (about 1-1/4 pounds total)

1/4 to 1/2 teaspoon black pepper

      Dash sea salt

1   teaspoon extra virgin olive oil

1/4 cup chicken broth

1   10-ounce package prewashed fresh spinach, trimmed (8 cups)

2   tablespoons walnut or pecan pieces, toasted

1   tablespoon lemon juice

      Lemon slices, halved (optional)

In a small bowl combine feta cheese and cream cheese; set aside. Using a sharp knife, cut a horizontal slit through the thickest portion of each chicken breast half to form a pocket. Stuff pockets with the cheese mixture. If necessary, secure openings with wooden toothpicks. Sprinkle chicken with pepper and salt.

In a large nonstick skillet cook chicken in hot oil over medium-high heat about 12 minutes or until tender and no longer pink, turning once (reduce heat to medium if chicken browns too quickly).

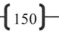

Remove chicken from skillet. Cover and keep warm.

Carefully add chicken broth to skillet. Bring to boiling; add half of the spinach. Cover and cook about 3 minutes or just until spinach is wilted. Remove spinach from skillet, reserving liquid in pan. Repeat with remaining spinach. Return all spinach to skillet. Stir in the nuts and lemon juice.

To serve, divide spinach mixture among 4 dinner plates. Top with chicken breasts. If desired, garnish with lemon slices.

*Note: If basil-and-tomato feta cheese is not available, stir 1 teaspoon finely snipped fresh basil and 1 teaspoon snipped oil-pack dried tomatoes, drained, into 1/4 cup plain feta cheese.

Nutrition Readout: 231 calories   FAT 8 g., PROTEIN 38 g., CARB 2 g., FIBER 6 g.

Thanksgiving Turkey with Low Carb Stuffing

Yes, Virginia, it is possible to create a low carb turkey stuffing that will taste just as good as grandmother's old fashioned made with biscuits, cornbread, and/or bread. The trick is to find a suitable substitute for all that forbidden starch.

Shirataki noodles are the answer.(you can order shiritaki noodles from www. Miracle Noodle.com or pick them up at your local Chinese grocery.) They're amazing. Calorie and carb free, they pick up the flavors around them, so when stuffed into the bird with all the other great veggies, it's just stupendous. Happy Turkey Day.

Because our celebration is small, I stuffed a turkey breast. You could also stuff a whole turkey, in which case, I would DOUBLE the stuffing ingredients. All good.

Makes 6-8 servings

1 5-pound boned and butterflied organic turkey breast with skin (get the butcher to do this)

Brine:

    1 cup kosher salt
    2 bay leaves
    3-4 peppercorns
    1/2 bottle white wine
    water to cover

Stuffing:

Extra virgin olive oil + butter to film the pan
1 large yellow onion, minced
3 celery ribs with leaves, minced

5 brown mushrooms chopped
1 pound sweet Italian sausage, removed from casing and crumbled
poultry seasoning + bay leaf
sea salt and cracked black pepper to taste
1 pound shirataki noodles, rinsed and chopped
1/2 cup walnut pieces
1/4 cup dried cranberries
2 large eggs, beaten

Begin brining the bird the day before. Add it to a large pan and add white wine, water to cover, and remaining ingredients. Cover and refrigerate overnight. Then, when you're ready to cook, remove to the counter and pat dry with paper towels.

Meanwhile, heat a 12-inch heavy skillet with olive oil and butter, then began sweating a large yellow onion, diced, then added diced celery and leaves a couple ribs, a bay leaf, sprinkled it with poultry seasoning and let it go a few minutes. While that is cooking over medium low heat, Peel 1 pound of Italian sweet sausage out of the skins and toss the meat into the skillet. Turn the fire up to brown the meat. Now chop 3-4 brown mushrooms and throw them in. Then a handful of walnuts, and a small amount of dried cranberries. It's beginning to look pretty good, but still lacks the "bulk" we think of.

So here's my bright idea for the day. Get out a one pound package of shiritaki noodles, rinse them, then cut the noodles with scissors and toss them into the mix, still letting it cook a bit. Adjust the seasonings with sea salt and cracked black pepper, Take it off heat to cool.

Finally beat a couple eggs and mix it with the cool stuffing ingredients.

Lay out the turkey breast and whack it some more with the pounder under wax paper until it was a uniform -- well sort of uniform - 1/2 inch thick. Spread the stuffing on top, leaving a narrow band around the edges Roll that sucker up, tie it with kitchen string three or four places and put it into a olive oiled Le Creuset baking dish.

Put it into a 375° degree oven, dab it with melted butter and let it roast until the thermometer registers 155 degrees. Whole kitchen smells great. Take it out. rest it a bit, cut and discard the strings, then take it to the table with accoutrement - green beans, Silver Cloud Cranberry Relish, and Fresh Pumpkin and Ginger Pickle. Yum.

Nutritional readout: 460 calories, FAT 34 g., Protein 35.6 g., carb 7.2 g, fiber 1.2 g.

Hotcha Flank Steak

Cook the whole thing in less than 10 minutes and feed 8 people once, or one person eight times.

Makes 8 servings

2 pounds flank steak
Kosher salt and cracked black pepper to taste
¼ cup fresh lime juice + grated zest from one lime
2 tablespoons extra virgin olive oil
6 cloves garlic, smashes
1 teaspoon (or to taste) crushed red pepper
½ teaspoon salt

Score flank steak and put it in a zip lock bag. Add remaining ingredients, zip it up and marinate. 30 minutes on the counter, up to 8 hours in the refrigerator. Heat grill and cook 4-5 minutes on each side. Rest on a cutting board, then cut into thin slices. Serve garnished with additional lime wedges.

Nutritional readout. 189 calories, FAT 8.9g. PROTEIN 24.8 g., CARB 1.3 g., FIBER 0.1 g.

Hoisin Beef Stir Fry with Asparagus and Red and Orange Bell Peppers

Just like going out to eat where you ask them to leave the rice to the side, this time, you'll just serve this in a bowl and enjoy it without any additional carbs.

Makes 6 servings ready to serve in less than 10 minutes

2 tablespoons soy sauce, divided
1 tablespoon cornstarch, divided
1 pound boneless beef steak, cut into ½ inch strips
½ cup chicken broth
2 tablespoons hoisin sauce
1 tablespoon rice vinegar
1 teaspoon dark sesame oil
¼ teaspoon crushed red pepper
¼ cup sesame oil, divided
1 red or orange bell pepper, sliced thin
1 pound asparagus, cut into 2-inch pieces\
1 green onion, thinly sliced
1 tablespoon sesame seeds, white or black

Combine half soy sauce and cornstarch in a bowl, whisk until smooth. Add beef, rubbing mixture into all surfaces.

Combine remaining soy, cornstarch, broth and hoisin, rice vinegar, dark oil, and red pepper. Heat 2 teaspoons sesame oil in a large skillet then sauté beef, stirring, about 5 minutes or until lightly browned. Remove to a warm bowl. Add remaining oil to skillet and stir fry the bell pepper, asparagus and green onion, until crisp tender. Add beef and broth mixture and cook until hot through, abut 30 seconds. Serve at once sprinkled with sesame seeds.

Nutritional readout: 243 calories, FAT 14.6 gm. PROTEIN 17.3 g, CARB 10.6 g., FIBER 2 g.

Stilton Beef with Sherry Mushroom Sauce

Got something to celebrate? Now you do. Add a side of roasted asparagus and it's a party.

Makes 4 4-ounce servings

4 4-ounce beef tenders (filet mignon)
Kosher salt and cracked black pepper to taste
2 tablespoons extra virgin olive oil
½ pound sliced mixed forest mushrooms
1 cup dry sherry
¼ cup Worcestershire
1 packet sugar substitute
1 teaspoon fresh oregano
1 ounce (1/4 cup) crumbled stilton (or other blue) cheese
¼ cup chopped fresh parsley

Season beef with salt and pepper. Heat a large skillet over medium high heat and sear steaks about 3 minutes per side for medium. Adding mushrooms once you've turned the meat. Meanwhile combine remaining ingredients except cheese in a bowl.

Remove steaks to a warm plate and cover. Add sherry mixture to the pan and reduce by half. Serve steaks with mushrooms and sauce. sprinkled with stilton.

Nutritional readout: 295 calories, FAT 11.3 g., PROTEIN 26 g., CARB 7.8 g., FIBER .8 g

Roast Pork Loin with Dry Cured Olives

Makes 10 servings.

Another dish that repays you with great leftovers for lunch, this luxurious looking dish is easy to prepare and rewarding to serve.

1 boneless pork loin (from 4 to 6 pounds)
½ cup seedless dry cured black olives
2 cloves garlic, slivered
1 teaspoon rosemary needles
Freshly milled black pepper to taste
1 tablespoon extra virgin olive oil
1 cup veal or beef stock
1 cup dry white wine
1cup pork skins, crushed
1 tablespoon Madeira

Heat oven to 400°. Cut deeply into the pork loin, lengthwise, to open up a flap. Then add olives, garlic, rosemary, and pepper. Roll and tie the roast at 1-inch intervals using cotton string. Heat oil in a large roasting pan in the oven, and then add the meat and brown for 15 minutes.

Meanwhile heat stock and wine, then pour over the meat, reduce heat to 325° and continue roasting until meat reaches an internal temperature of 140° Remove roast to a serving platter to rest. Add pork skins to pan juices and stir and boil to make a sauce. Add Madeira to sauce, then taste and adjust seasonings. Garnish with parsley. Slice thin and pass the gravy.

Nutritional readout: 422 calories, FAT 20.5 g., PROTEIN 48.8 g., CARB 5.3 g., FIBER .1 g

Pork Medallions in Capers

Choose boneless pork medallions for ease of use, or make thin slices from a pork tenderloin. This is on the table in less than ten minutes and may be served during the detox phase as well as the marathon.

Makes 4 servings

1 pound pork medallions
Kosher salt and freshly milled black pepper to taste
2 tablespoons extra virgin olive oil
¼ cup chicken broth
3 tablespoons capers, drained
2 tablespoons fresh lemon juice + grated zest of ½ lemon

Pound pork between wax paper to ¼-inch thickness. Season with salt and pepper. Heat oil in a large skillet over medium high heat, then cook pork, 2 minutes to the side, or until browned.

Add broth, capers, and lemon and cook 2-3 minutes, or until liquid has reduced by half. Serve hot.

Nutritional readout: 168 calories.   FAT 7.4 g., PROTEIN 23.3 g.,   CARB 1.3 g., FIBER .3 g.

Five Spice Lamb Chops with Raspberry Salsa

Quick as a wink and brightly flavored.

Makes 4 servings

8 trimmed lamb chops
2 teaspoons five spice powder
Salt and freshly milled black pepper to taste
2 cups fresh raspberries
1 teaspoon freshly grated ginger root
1 packet sugar substitute
2 teaspoons rice wine vinegar
2 tablespoons extra virgin olive oil

Season pork with five spice, salt and pepper. Combine raspberries, ginger, sugar substitute, and rice wine vinegar in a bowl.

Heat oil in a large skillet and cook meat, about 2 minutes to the side or until golden. Mound salsa over chops to serve.

Nutritional readout: 220 calories, FAT 9.2 g., PROTEIN 24 g., CARB 10 g., FIBER 1.7 g.

Parvathy Ramachandran's Egg Plant Chick Pea Gravy

Keep a pot of this luscious South Indian style sauce in the refrigerator and spoon it over cooked chicken or fish for a fantastic, flavorful one-dish dinner. Makes 10 servings

4 tablespoons olive or sesame oil (Choose sesame for the South Indian flavor)
1 tablespoon cumin seeds
1 teaspoon turmeric powder
1 large garlic clove, peeled and smashed
1 piece fresh ginger, about 1x2 inches, peeled and minced
½ small green or red hot pepper (optional) seeded, minced
1 small red onion, peeled and finely chopped
2 tablespoons garam masala OR madras curry powder dissolved in 2 tablespoons water
1 medium eggplant, chopped and salted with 1 teaspoon kosher salt
1 14-oz. can chopped tomatoes and juice
1 16-oz. can chickpeas, drained
½ cup fresh cilantro, chopped

Heat the fat in a large skillet then add cumin seeds and turmeric and allow to sputter; about 30 seconds, then add the garlic and ginger, along with the peppers. Add the onions and cook over medium heat, stirring, until the onion is clear, about 3 to 5 minutes. Add curry powder mixed in a little water. Stir vigorously, then add eggplant and cook until it begins to brown and soften, about 5 minutes. Add tomatoes and chickpeas and cook 10 minutes or so, tasting and adjusting salt as needed. Toss in cilantro at the end. Serve over meat, fish, or ¼ cup basmati rice, white or brown.

282 Cal, FAT 16.6 g, PROTEIN 25.1 g., CARB 8.2 g., FIBER 3.2 g

St. Croix Curry

The Indian Diaspora took curry to the Caribbean where it found a welcome home. You can almost hear the calypso beat when you cook this. Although goat is the meat of choice, you can substitute fish, veal, beef, lamb, or even chicken. The flavor is intense and satisfying. The work is minimal. You'll love it. Skip the traditional rice until you've come within 5 pounds of your goal weight.

Makes 8 servings

2 pounds boneless stew meat (veal, beef, lamb, chicken, or goat)
Kosher salt and freshly milled black pepper
2 tablespoons coconut oil (or olive oil)
1 large red onion, finely chopped
2 garlic cloves, crushed
1 tablespoon (or more to taste) hot curry powder
½ teaspoon ground cumin
½ teaspoon crushed red pepper (or to taste)
2 cups chicken broth
Juice and zest from 4 limes
½ cup minced green onions

Season meat generously with salt and pepper. Heat oil in a large deep stew pot, and then brown the meat, a few pieces at a time. Add onion and garlic and heat about a minute, then stir in curry powder, cumin, and red pepper. Heat another minute, then add broth and simmer until meat is tender, about an hour. Stir in lime juice and zest and serve topped with green onions. For those who have come within 5 pounds of goal weight, add ½ cup cooked brown rice to the bottom of your soup bowl and spoon curry on top.

Nutritional readout: 252 calories, FAT 15 g,, PROTEIN 24 g., CARB 5.2 g,, FIBER .9 g.

Kale With Garlic and Bacon

Quick to fix and deeply satisfying.

Makes 4 servings

1-1/2 pounds kale (about 2 bunches), tough stems and center ribs
cut off and discarded
10 bacon slices (1/2 pound), cut into 1/2-inch pieces
4 garlic cloves, finely chopped
½ teaspoon (or to taste) red chili flakes
1 cup chicken broth

Stack a few kale leaves and roll lengthwise into a cigar
shape. Cut crosswise into 1/4-inch-wide strips with a sharp knife.
Repeat with remaining leaves.

Cook bacon in a wide 6- to 8-quart heavy pot over
moderate heat, stirring occasionally, until crisp, then transfer with
a slotted spoon to paper towels to drain. Cook garlic and red chili
in remaining fat over moderately low heat, stirring, until pale
golden, about 30 seconds. Add kale (pot will be full) and cook,
turning with tongs, until wilted and bright green, about 1 minute.
Add broth and simmer, partially covered, until just tender, 6 to 10
minutes. Toss with bacon and salt and pepper to taste.

Nutritional Readout: 375 calories, FAT 26g; PROTEIN 22.31 g.,
CARBS 18.10 g., FIBER 1.36 g.

Bacon, Sausage and Cabbage Soup

The secret to the success of this soup is the method. Take your time, "sweat" the vegetables in order just until they have begun to glisten and turn brown before adding one drop of liquid and the flavor will simply leap out at you.

Makes 8 1-cup servings

4 strips thick bacon, chopped
1 6-inch piece link low fat kielbasa, cut into coins
3 celery sticks, thinly sliced
2 medium onions, thinly sliced
½ red or yellow bell pepper, thinly sliced
6 garlic cloves, thinly sliced
1 inch piece of fresh ginger, thinly sliced
1 tablespoon curry powder (or more to suit)
grated zest of one orange
1 small head Savoy or other cabbage, thinly sliced
Kosher salt and freshly ground black pepper to taste
1 quart chicken broth
1 14-1/2 oz. Can diced tomatoes and juice
Garnish: sour cream, minced cilantro and/or fresh jalapeno

In a large soup pot, over medium heat, begin to cook bacon and kielbasa. Meanwhile place slicing disk on the food processor and IN ORDER, begin slicing the vegetables. As you get each one sliced, add it to the pot.

Take your time. Let the vegetables cook down. Stir and don't rush. By the time you get to add the broth and tomatoes, the vegetables should have cooked down by half their volume. Once you've added the liquid, cover the pot and cook about 15 minutes.

Nutritional readout: 87 calories, FAT 4.7 g., PROTEIN 3.1 g, CARB 9.4 g., FIBER 2.4 g

Texas Caviar

Party fave for footballers, this healthy topping can lift a chicken breast, slice of pork roast or fish fillet to new heights.

Makes 20 ¼ cup servings

3 tablespoons chopped fresh cilantro
3 tablespoons red wine vinegar
2 tablespoons extra virgin olive oil
Hot sauce to taste, shake it on good
1 garlic clove, smashed
2 15.8 oz. cans black eyed peas, rinsed and drained
1-1/2 cups diced red onion
1 cup diced seeded tomato
1 cup diced red, green and/or yellow bell pepper

Toss all ingredients together in a large bowl. Cover and refrigerate.

Nutritional readout: 43 calories, FAT 1.6 g., PROTEIN 1.7 g. CARB 5.8 g., FIBER 1.4 g.

Summer Fruit Salsa

Spoon over no-sugar added ice cream or custard for a divine dessert.

Makes 12 ¼ cup servings

1-1/2 cups chopped cantaloupe
1 cup chopped pineapple
½ cup craisins (dried cranberries)
½ cup chopped fresh mint
2 tablespoons fresh lemon juice + grated zest from lemon
1 teaspoon grated fresh ginger root
1 small jalapeno, seeded and minced

Combine ingredients in a bowl, cover and refrigerate.

Nutritional Readout: 29 calories. FAT 0.1g. PROTEIN .3 g., CARB 7.7 g., FIBER .6 g

Bloody Mary Shrimp Dipper

OK. Go ahead and drink it out of the cup. It's that good and only 4.6 g. carbs per ¼ cup serving. But really, bathe cold boiled shrimp, oysters on the half shell or clams with this zesty flavor.

Makes 8 ¼ cup servings

1 cup thick Bloody Mary Cocktail mix
½ cup finely chopped sweet onion
½ cup minced cilantro
½ cup minced celery
½ cup chopped berry tomato
½ cup chopped celery leaves
Big shot of Worcestershire and Tabasco

Combine in a bowl, cover and refrigerate.

Nutritional readout: 20 calories, FAT .1g. PROTEIN .5 g., CARB 4.6 g., FIBER .8 g.

Index:

ORAL TESTIMONY TO THE USDA DIETARY GUIDELINES COMMITTEE
July 8, 2010

By Dr. John Salerno and Linda West Eckhardt, Founders – The Silver Cloud Diet

Presented to the USDA committee in a paper by Linda West Eckhardt

The proposed 2010 Dietary Guidelines continue the misguided shibboleths against saturated fats and animal foods rich in nutrient dense fatty acids, including egg yolks, butter, cream, whole milk, cheese and fatty meats including bacon as well as animal fats for cooking. In my 20 year practice of medicine in New York City, I have treated many patients whose health had been severely compromised by excluding these necessary nutrients in their daily diet. It is my experience, backed up by scientific studies, that low fat diets have caused many of today's lifestyle ailments including obesity, diabetes, heart disease and stroke.

Basic biochemistry shows that the human body has a high requirement for saturated fats in the cell membranes, brain and other organs. If we do not eat saturated fats, the body makes fat from refined carbohydrates, leading to rapid weight gain and chronic illness.

The proposed guidelines will exacerbate existing nutrient deficiencies that I see in my practice every day. Common deficiencies in vitamins A, D, K2 and E which are found in animal fats, vitamins B12 and B6, found in animal foods, as well as minerals including iron, calcium and zinc which require vitamins A and D for assimilation. It is my experience that these deficiencies can be easily corrected by a proper diet of whole foods, organic if possible, with naturally occurring animal fats. (give anecdote here)

I have seen, in my practice, children as young as 8 years old, suffering from type 2 diabetes, an ailment that used to be seen only in later middle age. Why are these children getting diabetes? Low fat milk, soy milk, apple juice, too many processed carbohydrates, and insufficient natural animal fats. Fortunately, type 2 diabetes can be stopped in its tracks by a radical shift in the diet. Give those children whole milk, plenty of protein and natural animal fats, get the sugars out of their diets, and their diabetes will correct itself, their weight will normalize and they will be healthy.

Our misguided dietary public policy has created a society of very sick people. For the first time in history we see a generation who may not live as long as its parents.

Particularly in the lower classes without access to healthy, whole foods, we are creating a society of people who will not be well, who will require huge public assistance and health care, and all of it could be alleviated by a proper diet.

From the viewpoint of a practicing physician, I can tell you that our industrial food complex, in concert with big pharma have colluded to create a society where people eat nutrient-empty processed foods, and are than given an ever larger regimen of pharmaceuticals to try and turn back the inevitable ill health and death that awaits them.

Besides the fact that our enormously powerful industrial food/farming lobby has exercised great control over public policy for at least twenty years, since I have been observing it, the results, in the time that I have been practicing medicine, have been dreadful.

When I was a boy, growing up in an Italian American family, my grandfather had a big vegetable garden out back that fed our family. He lived to be 95 years old and was strong and active until the day he died. I try to feed my family, whole, organic foods to this day. My six year old son, rides with me in bicycle races for as much as 45 miles at a time. This child is healthy, vigorous, and cheerful. He gets whole milk, plenty of butter and red meat, and a good assortment of whole organic fruits and vegetables.

Is it impossible that Americans could eat as well as their grandparents? Not at all. With the growing movement towards healthier whole foods being presented not only at home, but in public schools, institutions, and food service operations, Americans are beginning to get it.

At The Silver Cloud Diet we particularly recognize the need for saturated fats, for health, long life, and weight loss. Saturated fats fight inflammation, support the immune system, support hormone production and protect against cancer and heart disease.

Last but not least what I see in my practice that is most heartbreaking is the rising tide of infertility. Now that we have an entire generation of young women who have practically grown up eating a low fat diet, we see a pandemic of infertility. The simple truth is that vitamins carried in saturated animal fats are critical to reproduction. The 2010 Guidelines proposed by the USDA will increase infertility in this country. This is tragic and entirely avoidable.

The knee-jerk recommendation to eat more whole grains, does not take into account the fact that whole grains are extremely difficult to digest and an overconsumption of rough whole grains can contribute to digestive disorders such as celiac disease and irritable bowel syndrome.

The Silver Cloud Diet recommends that people eat a diet of whole, unprocessed foods, organic if possible, that provide an abundance of nutrients chosen from the following groups:

1. Animal foods: meat and organ meats, poultry and eggs from pastured animals, wild caught fish and shell fish, whole raw cheeses, milk and other dairy products from pastured animals.
2. Fats and oils: unrefined saturated and monounsaturated fats including butter, lard, olive oil, cod liver oil and coconut and palm oil.
3. Fruits and Vegetables. Fresh, organic if possible, preferably locally grown, either raw or cooked into soups and stews
4. Nuts, legumes, and grains. Eat a handful of nuts daily for vitamin E and trace minerals. Once goal weight is reached eat beans and lentils, brown rice, and whole grain cooked cereals for breakfast.

We do not recommend processed foods with long lists of ingredient including chemicals you cannot pronounce. No refined sweeteners including candy, soda, cookies, crackers, cakes, chips or other snacks. Avoid white flour products such as pasta and white bread. Avoid processed foods including modern soy foods, polyunsaturated and partially hydrogenated vegetable oils and fried foods.

As we say at the Silver Cloud Diet, take a giant leap backwards. Eat the way your grandparents ate. You take care of your body and your body will take care of you.

Index

Recipe Index

Marathon Recipes:
Meat

Poultry

Seafood

Vegetable

Biographies of the authors

Dr. John P. Salerno, Board Certified, American Boards of Family Practice

Lauded as an international pioneer in the field of anti-aging, Dr. John P. Salerno is a leader in the practice of complementary medicine. Based in Manhattan, Dr. Salerno has been cited as an expert by national media outlets, retained as a consultant by world-renowned medical luminaries for the launching of treatment facilities across three continents, and referenced by Suzanne Somers in her #1 New York Times bestseller, Ageless, and in her 2009 follow-ups, Breakthrough and Knockout. Somers told an audience in 2006, "I will personally send patients to Dr. Salerno."

Dr. Salerno is the founder of the Salerno Center for Complementary Medicine established in New York City in 2005. He is also the co-founder of anti-aging clinics in Tokyo; the chief medical officer behind the RenuLife anti-aging and dermatological clinic in Sao Paolo, Brazil.

Best known for his weight-loss treatments, bio-identical hormone replacement, vitamin IV suites, and chelation therapy, a process that removes heavy metals from the body, Dr. Salerno lists dozens of celebrities among his patients. He combines the teachings of traditional medicine with the wisdom of alternative healing to cleanse the system of toxins and blockages that can cause heart disease, cancer, brain dysfunction, diabetes and others. He boosts the body's immune system with products chosen from a line of natural vita-nutrients that he created in conjunction with Dr. Hiroyuki Abe, president of The International Society of Integrative Medicine and owner of the Kudan Clinic in Japan.

Dr. Salerno is a licensed physician in the State of New York and in Florida. He is also a diplomate of the National Board of

Osteopathic Medical Examiners, a board certified member of the American Osteopathic Board of Family Practice and member in good standing of the American Osteopathic Association, the American College for Advancement in Medicine, the American Medical Association and the American Academy of Anti-Aging Medicine.

Dr. Salerno graduated magna cum laude from Adelphi University, where he earned a Bachelor of Science in Biology, and received his Doctor of Osteopathic Medicine degree from New York College of Osteopathic Medicine of New York Institute of Technology. He completed his internship and Family Practice residency at New York's Long Beach Medical Center, during which time he conducted lab research at the Columbia University Medical Center.

Linda West Eckhardt, is an award winning journalist, food writer, and nutritionist. Her more than 20 cookbooks have garnered prizes including the James Beard prize for the best cookbook for a book she wrote with her daughter, Katherine West DeFoyd, entitled ***Entertaining 101.*** Doubleday. Their follow-up book, ***Stylish One Dish Dinners***, Doubleday, was also nominated for a James Beard prize. Their next book, ***The High Protein Cookbook,*** Clarkson Potter, remains a best seller after 12 years. That book was designed to accompany low carb diet plans. Her ground-breaking book, ***Bread in Half The Time***, Broadway Books, was named the Best Cookbook in American by the prestigious IACP, The Julia Child award. Her award winning radio work with Jennifer English, for a national show on the Food and Wine radio network, was nominated for a James Beard Prize for a show called, ***"I Know What You Ate Last Summer."***

Ms. Eckhardt has published hundreds of magazine pieces in national magazines, was a food columnist for Cooking Light Magazine, The Oregonian, Texas Monthly, and the Grants Pass Courier. She holds a Bachelors' degree in foods and nutrition from The University of Texas, and a Masters' degree in English,

Creative Writing, from San Francisco State University, both with honors.

She has published a baker's dozen short stories, written two novels, and had one optioned to the movies. Her food essays have appeared in journals for more than 20 years.

Never one to shy away from progress, Ms. Eckhardt has leapt into the digital age and become something of an expert on content provision for the internet, as well an expert and successful blogger on sites including Amy Ephron's *One for The Table,* Jeff Deasy's *American Feast,* and is co-founder of the successful *The Silver Cloud Diet*, where she continues to create daily content, test and offer recipes, and provide a bird's eye view of the low-carb diet revolution occurring in the U.S.

She was invited to present testimony at the USDA hearings for the New Food Pyramid, in Summer, 2010. In addition, she travels the world learning about food patterns, as well as traditional and new foods. She takes select friends to Italy annually for a food and wine tour.

Her new book, *Skinny Girl Cocktails,* is in process.